Worlds
of
Experience

Also by Robert Stolorow, Donna Orange, and George Atwood
Working Intersubjectively

Also by Robert Stolorow and George Atwood
Contexts of Being
Faces in a Cloud
Structures of Subjectivity
Psychoanalytic Treatment

Also by Donna Orange
Emotional Understanding: Studies in Psychoanalytic Epistemology

Worlds of Experience

Interweaving Philosophical and Clinical Dimensions in Psychoanalysis

Robert D. Stolorow
George E. Atwood
Donna M. Orange

BASIC
BOOKS

A Member of the Perseus Books Group

Copyright © 2002 by Robert D. Stolorow, George E. Atwood, Donna M. Orange

Published by Basic Books,
A Member of the Perseus Books Group

Designed by Reginald Thompson

Library of Congress Cataloging-in-Publication Data
Stolorow, Robert D.
    Worlds of experience : interweaving philosophical and clinical dimensions in psychoanalysis / Robert D. Stolorow, George E. Atwood, Donna M. Orange.
    p. cm.
    Includes bibliographical references and index.
    ISBN 0-465-09574-7 (alk. paper)
    1. Psychoanalysis. I. Atwood, George E. II. Orange, Donna M. III. Title.
RC504.S763 2003
616.89'17—dc21
2002010825

03 04 / 10 9 8 7 6 5 4 3 2 1

Contents

I hold in my hand the world.
    —Emily Stolorow (age six)

Preface

Over the course of nearly three decades, our intersubjective systems perspective has evolved from early studies of the subjective origins of psychoanalytic theories (Stolorow and Atwood, 1979) into a phenomenological field theory (Atwood and Stolorow, 1984) and perspectivalist (Orange, 1995), contextualist sensibility (Orange, Atwood, and Stolorow, 1997) with rich implications for a broad array of psychoanalytic clinical questions (Stolorow, Brandchaft, and Atwood, 1987) and for a radical rethinking of the basic pillars of psychoanalytic theory (Stolorow and Atwood, 1992). This book penetrates to the philosophical underpinnings of both psychoanalytic theory and practice. Our aim here is twofold: first, to expose and deconstruct the assumptions, largely a legacy of Descartes's philosophy, that have undergirded traditional and much contemporary psychoanalytic thinking; and second, to lay the foundations for a post-Cartesian psychoanalytic psychology grounded in intersubjective contextualism.

We begin, in Chapter 1, with an exploration of the personal and relational contexts in which Descartes's philosophy took form, as well as a demonstration of how a focus on affectivity recontextualizes virtually all facets of the Cartesian isolated mind. Chapter 2 shows how the shift from Cartesian to post-Cartesian thinking in psychoanalysis entails a move away from isolated minds and toward experiential worlds as its central theoretical and clinical focus. The three theoretical chapters that follow (Chapters 3–5) illuminate the hidden Cartesian, isolated-mind assumptions that saturate Freudian, Kohutian self-psychological, and contemporary relational theorizing, and they offer a post-Cartesian alternative to the Freudian unconscious rooted in intersubjective systems theory. Chapters 6–8 illustrate the profound clinical implications of adopting a post-Cartesian, contextualist perspective—for the ambience of the psychoanalytic situation and for the understanding and therapeutic approach to states of severe psychological trauma and experiences of personal annihilation.

Chapter 3 was first published in *Contemporary Psychoanalysis* (2001, vol. 37(1), pp. 43–61). Substantial portions of Chapters 2, 4, 5, 7, and 8 were previously published in *Psychoanalytic Psychology* (1999, vol. 16, pp. 380–388 and 464–468; 2001, vol. 18, pp. 287–302, 380–387, and 468–484; 2002, vol. 19, pp. 281–306). We are grateful to the editors and publishers of these journals for granting us permission to include this material in our book.

1

Introduction:
Contextualizing Descartes
and the Isolated Mind

I think, therefore I am.
> —René Descartes

When [human Being] directs itself towards
something and grasps it, it does not somehow
first get out of an inner sphere in which it has
been proximally encapsulated, but its primary
kind of Being is such that it is always "outside"
alongside entities which it encounters and
which belong to a world already discovered. . .
[A] bare subject without a world never "is"
. . . .

> —Martin Heidegger

The assumptions of traditional psychoanalysis have been pervaded by the Cartesian doctrine of the isolated mind. This doctrine bifurcates the subjective world of the person into outer and inner regions, reifies and absolutizes the resulting separation between the two, and pictures the mind as an objective entity that takes its place among other objects, a "thinking thing" that has an inside with contents and looks out on an external world from which it is essentially estranged.

Since the publication of the first edition of *Faces in a Cloud* (Stolorow and Atwood, 1979), our own approach has been a post-Cartesian, phenomenological one, focused on worlds of individual experience. Phenomenology, although owing much to Descartes in its origin, seeks knowledge of experience in its own distinctively subjective terms, avoiding concepts that objectify consciousness by localizing it within a mind, psyche, or psychical apparatus of any kind. Experience or consciousness, from a phenomenological point of view, is immaterial and nonsubstantial, which means it has none of the properties that belong to material things, such as location in space, momentum, causal efficacy, and the like. As our own thinking has gradually evolved from our early proposals for a "psychoanalytic phenomenology" (Stolorow and Atwood, 1979; Atwood and Stolorow, 1984) into a fully intersubjective systems theory (Stolorow and Atwood, 1992; Orange, Atwood, and Stolorow, 1997), we have noted that we are often misunderstood as promoting a radical subjectivism and relativism. This misreading, we believe, arises because of a continuing commitment of so many in our field to the Cartesian doctrine of the isolated mind, a standpoint from which the ideas and clinical descriptions of intersubjectivity theory inevitably appear elusive, like quicksilver, as if one were operating in some imaginary space lacking all definite form and substance. These impressions are not generated by any special subtlety or complexity inhering in the intersubjective approach as such; it is rather that unexamined Cartesian assumptions produce an illusion of solidity and definiteness in psychological thinking, and when those assumptions are suspended, the result can be a subjective effect of confusion, ambiguity, and even anxiety (Bernstein, 1983). Suddenly, the mind and the stable external world pictured as surrounding it lose their status as absolutes, and psychoanalytic observation and theory, now concerned solely with experience and its organization, no longer appear to be anchored in anything solidly real.

In *Contexts of Being* (Stolorow and Atwood, 1992), we raised this question: Why is it that the doctrine of the isolated mind, so manifestly a hindrance to the development of psychoanalytic understanding, has nevertheless maintained such a tenacious hold on thinkers in our field? We addressed the question by proposing that this doctrine is actually a myth of our culture, an illusory, alienating image of our own existence that serves to shield us from a sense of "the unbearable embeddedness of being" (p. 22), that is, from an excruciating feeling of our own human finiteness, dependency, and mortality. By holding to the notion that each of us is essentially a solitary, self-contained unit, we are specifically protected from an otherwise intolerable feeling of vulnerability to the human surround.

We now return to the life and ideas of René Descartes himself, to try to better grasp his original formulations of this doctrine and the psychological sources of its persistent hold on our field. Reading through Descartes's classic essays *Discourse on Method* ([1637] 1989a) and *Meditations* ([1641] 1989b), one sees a search for a reliable and certain foundation for philosophy and all human knowledge, a truth so incontestably solid that it could provide a starting point for the rebuilding of the sciences

on a basis of unassailable validity. Descartes followed a
method of systematic doubt, progressively setting aside
each of his convictions that could not be established as
self-evidently true, until he finally arrived at the one that
could be so established: "I think, therefore I am" *(cogito
ergo sum)*. Each of us is, according to his argument,
assured of the fact of our own existence by virtue of our
thinking itself, and this provides the one certain foundation on which everything else we may securely believe
must be based. But what exactly is it that Descartes's systematic doubt has supposedly revealed us to be? He said
that each of us is a mind, a thinking thing, a thing that is
certain of its own singular existence but of nothing else.
As we watch Descartes's thought experiment, we see with
Cartesian clarity how much the standpoint of the
observer influences the observations that are made and
the conclusions that are reached. An isolated observer
turns inward in the search for something secure and certain, and he discovers the existence of his own isolated
mind. This doctrine of mind that has so pervasive a presence in psychoanalysis and in our culture generally is
Cartesian philosophy transformed by history into common sense.

The Cartesian mind, almost immediately after being
"discovered" through the method of systematic doubt,
begins to undergo a reification, that is, a conversion into
an objective entity that takes its place among other
objects. Although Descartes told us that the mind lacks
the property of extension in space possessed by material
bodies, he nevertheless called it a "thinking thing" and
moreover located psychological faculties as existing somehow "inside" it. In addition, as he developed ideas about

the relation of mind and body, he pictured the mind as an entity that enters into causal interaction with physical objects. So the mind is a thing, a thing with an inside, and furthermore it enters into causal interaction with other physical entities. How might one psychologically understand the original elaboration of this doctrine that has had such a fateful influence on us all? Why would a man need to find an absolutely reliable and certain foundation for what he believed, something about which he could never be deceived? And why did the solution he discovered take the form of a reified concept of the existence of his own solitary selfhood?

Some scholars have sought answers to such questions through an analysis of the social and historical context of Descartes's thought (Bernstein, 1983; Toulmin, 1990; Gaukroger, 1995; Slavin, 2002), pointing to extreme instability in the political, intellectual, and religious spheres of life. Surely the Cartesian quest for certainty must be viewed against the backdrop of a European historical situation during the seventeenth century involving challenges to traditional structures of faith, revolutionary understandings of the human place in the cosmos (Copernicus, Galileo), and political crises and decades of warfare threatening the stability of life for everyone. Here, however, we seek the context of the Cartesian quest in Descartes's individual life and history, for his search must also have had its sources within its originator's unique personal experiences.

It is difficult to understand much of the life of someone who was born 400 years ago and who in addition was suspicious of others and extremely secretive about all personal things (Gaukroger, 1995). Descartes was born in

1596, into a family consisting of his father, an official working for the French Parliament, his mother, and two older siblings. Descartes's mother died when he was thirteen months old, whereupon his father sent him to live with his maternal grandmother, along with his brother and sister. At age ten, he was sent to a Jesuit college, where he boarded for the next seven years. When he was fourteen, his grandmother died as well. The biographer Stephen Gaukroger described Descartes as having had a persistent tendency toward melancholia and paranoia, linking this disposition to the loss of his mother and his home, and to the later separation from and loss of his grandmother. Could these early upheavals in his life have been the source of his lifelong need for something unassailably certain, something that would be absolutely solid and secure? In Descartes's philosophy, certainty and security are finally found, not in relationships with other human beings but rather in the isolated workings of his own mind, envisioned as a rational, self-contained, self-sufficient entity.

In an importantly revealing letter to Princess Elizabeth of Bohemia, for whom Descartes served as a personal adviser and confessor, at times almost as a psychotherapist, he discussed an illness from which she was suffering—what he called a "slow fever"—that in his view was caused by "sadness." He recommended a form of mental discipline in which the imagination is directed away from the reasons for distress and toward "consideration of objects which could furnish contentment and joy," thereby "free[ing] her mind from all sad thoughts" (Cottingham et al., 1991, p. 250). He then went on to say something very interesting about himself:

I take the liberty of adding that I found by experience in my own case that the remedy I have suggested cured an illness almost exactly similar, and perhaps even more dangerous . . . My mother died a few days [!] after my birth from a disease of the lung caused by distress. From her I inherited a dry cough and a pale colour which stayed with me until I was more than twenty, so that all the doctors who saw me up to that time condemned me to die young. But I have always had an inclination to look at things from the most favourable angle and *to make my principal happiness depend upon myself alone*, and I think this inclination caused the indisposition, which was almost part of my nature, gradually to disappear. (Cottingham et al., 1991, pp. 250–251, emphasis added)

Reflecting on the content of the letters from which this passage is drawn, one sees that Descartes was writing about physical conditions rooted in sadness as their primary cause, conditions that, as he said, were "almost part of my nature." He sought to overcome this "indisposition" by making his principal happiness depend upon himself alone. The proneness to depression and sadness resulting from the losses incurred in early life highlight the vulnerability of a man who could not find security and well-being through connections to the human world outside of himself, and who was driven instead to find contentment and peace on the terrain of his own inner soul.

Descartes's letters bear many further signs of the theme of self-reliance and especially of his belief that one's sense of well-being in the face of adversity is always to be secured through the use of one's own rational mind. In a letter to Constantijn Huygens (father of the physicist Christian Huygens), Descartes addressed his friend's feelings of grief and sorrow about the hopeless situation and impending death of a beloved companion. He told Huygens that he need not continue in a state of suffering because reason can overcome grief, and since Huygens was a man whose "life is governed entirely in accordance with reason," he should have no difficulty regaining his former peace of mind now that he knew "all hope of remedy has gone . . . " (Cottingham et al., 1991, p. 54). In another letter to Princess Elizabeth, Descartes extolled the virtue of becoming detached from the passions (that is, intense affects) and from the pleasures of the body, because they inevitably involve us with the world of transitory things. True happiness, according to his discussion, is to be found not in the "passing joys which depend upon the senses" but rather in an inner consciousness, "a mental satisfaction and contentment" in which one guards against "the false appearances of the goods of this world" by devoting oneself to the more lasting "pleasures . . . of the soul" (Cottingham et al., 1991, p. 267). Vulnerability to suffering occasioned by loss is thus overcome through a turning away from attachments to the transitory objects of the external world and toward a contemplative rationality seated in the inner recesses of one's own mind.

Seeking solace and comfort in the privacy of his own thinking, Descartes tried to distract himself from the "exquisite vulnerability accompanying an unalienated awareness of the continual embeddedness of human experience in constitutive intersubjective [that is, relational] context" (Stolorow and Atwood, 1992, p. 22). Thus, in the personal context of Descartes's life, at the very point of origin of the doctrine of the isolated mind, there appear vivid signs of the disavowal of one's dependence on and emotional vulnerability to others that this doctrine so pervasively and relentlessly expresses.

We would contrast the solitary reflection that led to Descartes's philosophical ideas with the dialogue out of which our intersubjective approach was born. The process by which intersubjectivity theory has developed since the 1970s necessarily mirrors and expresses the central concept around which this point of view has come into being. The idea of the intersubjective field, understood as a system of interacting, differently organized subjective worlds, emerged from the intersection of the various personal and intellectual perspectives each of the participants brought to the ongoing collaboration. Far from being the brainchild of any single individual, our viewpoint crystallized out of a shared enterprise of rethinking foundational concepts in psychoanalysis in the light of a thoroughgoing, self-reflexive contextualism.

Within philosophy, perhaps the most important challenge to the Cartesian isolated mind and subject-object split was mounted by Heidegger ([1927] 1962). In striking contrast to Descartes's detached, worldless subject, for Heidegger the Being of human life was primordially embedded and engaged "in-the-world." In Heidegger's vision, human Being is saturated with the world in which it dwells, just as the inhabited world is drenched in human meanings and purposes. In view of this fundamental contextualization, Heidegger's consideration of affect is especially noteworthy.

Heidegger's word for affectivity (feelings and moods) is *Befindlichkeit*, a characteristically cumbersome noun he invented to capture a basic dimension of human existence. Literally, the word might be translated as "how-one-finds-oneself-ness." As Eugene Gendlin (1988) has pointed out, Heidegger's word for affectivity denotes both how one feels and the situation within which one is feeling, a felt sense of oneself in a situation, prior to a Cartesian split between inside and outside. For Heidegger, *Befind-lichkeit*—affectivity—is a mode of living, of being-in-the-world, profoundly embedded in constitutive context. Heidegger's concept underscores the exquisite context-dependence and context-sensitivity of human emotional life.

Descartes's philosophy not only segregated inner from outer and subject from object; it also severed mind from body and cognition (reason) from affect. As seen in the biographical vignettes cited earlier, Descartes assigned to reason the task of overcoming and subjugating painful affect (like sadness), which he viewed as a source of physical illness. Correspondingly, the elevation of reason and the denigration of affective life are inherent features of his doctrine of the isolated mind. In contrast, affect—that is, subjective emotional experience—has become a center-piece of our psychoanalytic framework.

It is our contention that a shift in psychoanalytic thinking from the primacy of drive to the primacy of affectivity moves psychoanalysis toward a phenomenological contextualism (Orange, Atwood, and Stolorow, 1997) and a central focus on dynamic intersubjective systems (Stolorow, 1997). Unlike drives, which originate deep within the interior of a Cartesian isolated mind, affect is something that from birth onward is regulated, or misregulated, within ongoing relational systems. Therefore, locating affect at its center automatically entails a radical contextualization of virtually all aspects of human psychological life.

Our systematic focus on affectivity began with an early article written with Daphne Socarides Stolorow (Socarides and Stolorow, 1984–1985), attempting to integrate our evolving intersubjective perspective with the framework of Kohutian self psychology. In a proposed expansion and refinement of Heinz Kohut's (1971) selfobject concept, the authors suggested that "selfobject functions pertain fundamentally to the integration of affect" into the organization of self-experience and that the need for selfobject ties "pertains most centrally to the need for [attuned] responsiveness to affect states in all stages of the life cycle" (p. 105). Kohut's discussions of the longing for mirroring, for example, were seen as pointing to the role of appreciative attunement in the integration of expansive affect states, whereas his descriptions of the idealizing yearning were seen as indicating the importance of attuned emotional holding and containment in the integration of painful reactive affect states. In this early article, emotional experience was grasped as being inseparable from the intersubjective contexts of attunement and malattunement in which it was felt.

Numerous studies in developmental psychology and even neurobiology have affirmed the central motivational importance of affective experience as it is constituted relationally within child-caregiver systems (see Sander, 1985; Stern, 1985; Demos and Kaplan, 1986; Lichtenberg, 1989; Beebe and Lachmann, 1994; Jones, 1995; Brothers, 1997; Siegel, 1999). Grasping the motivational primacy of affectivity—*Befindlichkeit*—enables us to contextualize a wide range of psychological phenomena that have traditionally been the focus of psychoanalytic inquiry, including psychic conflict, trauma, transference and resistance, unconsciousness, and the therapeutic action of psychoanalytic interpretation.

The early article on affects and selfobject functions (Socarides and Stolorow, 1984–1985) alluded to the nature of the intersubjective contexts in which psychological conflict takes form: "An absence of steady, attuned responsiveness to the child's affect states leads to . . . significant derailments of optimal affect integration and to a propensity to dissociate or disavow affective reactions" (p. 106). Psychological conflict develops when central affect states of the child cannot be integrated because they evoke massive or consistent malattunement from caregivers (Stolorow, Brandchaft, and Atwood, 1987, chap. 6). Such unintegrated affect states become the source of lifelong emotional conflict and vulnerability to traumatic states because they are experienced as threats both to the person's established psychological organization and to the maintenance of vitally needed ties. Defenses against affect thus become necessary.

From this perspective, developmental trauma is viewed not as an instinctual flooding of an ill-equipped Cartesian container but as an experience of unbearable affect. Furthermore, the intolerability of an affect state cannot be explained solely, or even primarily, on the basis of the quantity or intensity of the painful feelings evoked by an injurious event. Traumatic affect states can be grasped only in terms of the relational systems in which they are felt (Stolorow and Atwood, 1992, chap. 4). Developmental trauma originates within a formative intersubjective context whose central feature is malattunement to painful affect—a breakdown of the child-caregiver system of mutual regulation—leading to the child's loss of affect-integrating capacity and thereby to an unbearable, over-whelmed, disorganized state. Painful or frightening affect becomes traumatic when the attunement that the child needs to assist in its tolerance, containment, and modulation is profoundly absent.

One consequence of developmental trauma, relationally conceived, is that affect states take on enduring, crushing meanings. From recurring experiences of malattunement, the child acquires the unconscious conviction that unmet developmental yearnings and reactive painful feeling states are manifestations of a loathsome defect or of an inherent inner badness. A defensive self-ideal is often established, representing a self-image purified of the offending affect states that were perceived to be unwelcome or damaging to caregivers. Living up to this affectively purified ideal becomes a central requirement for maintaining harmonious ties to others and for upholding self-esteem. Thereafter, the emergence of prohibited affect is experienced as a failure to embody the required ideal, an exposure of the underlying essential defectiveness or badness, and is accompanied by feelings of isolation, shame, and self-loathing. In the psychoanalytic situation, qualities or activities of the analyst that lend themselves to being interpreted according to such unconscious meanings of affect confirm the patient's expectations in the transference that emerging feeling states will be met with disgust, disdain, disinterest, alarm, hostility, withdrawal, exploitation, and the like or will damage the analyst and destroy the therapeutic bond. Such transference expectations, unwittingly confirmed by the analyst, are a powerful source of resistance to the experience and articulation of affect. Intractable repetitive transferences and resistances can be grasped, from this perspective, as rigidly stable "attractor states" (Thelen and Smith, 1994) of the patient-analyst system, in which the meanings of the analyst's style have become tightly coordinated with the patient's grim expectations and fears, thereby exposing the patient repeatedly to threats of retraumatization. The focus on affect and its meanings contextualizes both transference and resistance.

A second consequence of developmental trauma is a severe constriction and narrowing of the horizons of emotional experiencing, so as to exclude whatever feels unacceptable, intolerable, or too dangerous in particular intersubjective fields. Chapter 3 details how the focus on affect contextualizes the so-called repression barrier—the very boundary between conscious and unconscious. *Befindlichkeit* includes both feeling and the contexts in which it is or is not permitted to come into being.

Like constricted and narrowed horizons of emotional experiencing, expanding horizons too can only be grasped in terms of the intersubjective contexts within which they take form. We conclude this introduction with some remarks about the therapeutic action of psychoanalytic interpretation.

There has been a long-standing debate in psychoanalysis over the role of cognitive insight versus affective attachment in the process of therapeutic change. The terms of this debate are directly descended from

Descartes's philosophical dualism, which sectioned human experience into cognitive and affective domains. Such artificial fracturing of human subjectivity is no longer tenable in a post-Cartesian philosophical world. Cognition and affect, thinking and feeling, interpreting and relating—these are separable only in pathology, as we have seen in the case of Descartes himself, the profoundly isolated man who created a doctrine of the isolated mind, of disembodied, unembedded, decontextualized *cogito*.

The dichotomy between insight through interpretation and affective bonding with the analyst is revealed to be a false one, once we recognize that the therapeutic impact of analytic interpretations lies not only in the insights they convey but also in the extent to which they demonstrate the analyst's attunement to the patient's affective life. We have long contended that a good (that is, a mutative) interpretation is a relational process, a central constituent of which is the patient's experience of having his or her feelings understood (Stolorow, Atwood, and Ross, 1978). Furthermore, it is the specific transference meaning of the experience of being understood that supplies its mutative power (Stolorow, [1993] 1994), as the patient weaves that experience into the tapestry of developmental longings mobilized by the analytic engagement. Interpretation does not stand apart from the emotional relationship between patient and analyst; it is an inseparable, crucial dimension *of* that relationship. In the language of intersubjective systems theory, interpretive expansion of the patient's capacity for reflective awareness of old, repetitive organizing principles or emotional convictions occurs concomitantly with the affective impact and meanings of ongoing relational experiences with the analyst, and both are indissoluble components of a unitary therapeutic process that establishes the possibility of alternative principles for organizing experience, whereby the patient's emotional horizons can become widened, enriched, more flexible, and more complex. For this developmental process to be sustained, the analytic bond must be able to withstand the painful and frightening affect states that can accompany cycles of destabilization and reorganization (Stolorow, 1997). Clearly, a clinical focus on affective experience within the intersubjective field of an analysis contextualizes the process of therapeutic change in multiple ways. We turn now to a central theoretical idea with profoundly contextualizing implications—the concept of an experiential world.

Part One

Theoretical Studies

2

From Cartesian Minds
to Experiential Worlds

Mind is social and society is mental.
—Ian Suttie

O world! world! world! thus is the poor agent despised.
—William Shakespeare

Being-in-the-world, as concern, is fascinated by the world *with which it is concerned....* *[U]nderstanding of [one's] existence as such is always an understanding of the world.*
—Martin Heidegger

One of us recently overheard a colleague making a categorical statement to the effect that philosophy is useless, an occupation for dilettantes. "Now, psychoanalytic therapy," he continued, "there's something practical. Sometimes people really do need that." We could hope that despite Freud's well-known aversion to philosophy, most psychoanalysts today would not respond in this way, understanding that the inquiries and disputes of philosophers have something very important to do with their work. A sign that such understanding is indeed becoming more prevalent is the critical discussion of "Cartesianism" that has been occurring for the past decade in our field. In this chapter, offered as a further contribution to this discussion, we provide a list of the essential Cartesian ideas that have found their way into the theory and practice of psychoanalysis. We are indebted to the writings of philosopher Charles Taylor (1989) for this highly schematized account. (Consulting Taylor's richly nuanced work in the history of ideas will make it clear that he is not responsible for our simplifications. Even less is he responsible for what some readers may experience as a caricature of traditional psychoanalytic work. Clearly, the best analysts have always worked relationally, beyond the Cartesian framework, no matter what their official theoretical commitments.)

The Cartesian mind, in its origins familiar to many of us from early readings of Descartes's ([1641] 1989b) *Meditations,* developed over the modern era into the mental mechanism we know in the work of Freud. Although Freud's systematic study of unconscious processes undermined an important component of the Cartesian mind, namely, its devotion to "clear and distinct ideas," the psychoanalytic mind, as Marcia Cavell (1991, 1993) has masterfully shown, has been and continues to be the Cartesian mind. For most of us, the entire complex of presuppositions that we are calling the Cartesian mind is largely unconscious, embedded in the underlying grammar of our Western languages, and continues to characterize our psychoanalytic thinking and work. We think, therefore, that this form of psychoanalytic and philosophical unconsciousness deserves our continuing attention.

The Cartesian mind, including its positivist and empiricist variants, has several important qualities, each of which has bearing on our psychoanalytic work. (By "positivist" we mean antimetaphysical and devoted to verification and repeatability of experiment as knowledge criteria. The unrepeatability of the human individual makes this form of positivism unsuited for understanding the psychoanalytic process.) Let us briefly outline these qualities of the Cartesian mind, comparing them and their psychoanalytic consequences with those of experiential or psychological worlds. Our intent is not to engage in "outing" closet Cartesians—all of us, at times, would have to be included—but rather to make it easier for analysts to say more exactly what they are claiming and criticizing when they call themselves "post-Cartesians." In this spirit, we speak of ideas and their practical consequences, not so much of theorists, whom we see as conversation partners, fellow members of the community of inquirers. Our attempt here is to outline an alternative way of thinking and hint at its fruitfulness for psychoanalytic thinking and work.

The Cartesian Mind

First, self-enclosed isolation is the quality of psychological Cartesianism that we have already most extensively addressed. In *Working Intersubjectively* (Orange, Atwood, and Stolorow, 1997), we wrote:

An objectivist epistemology envisions the mind in isolation, radically separated from an external reality that it either accurately apprehends or distorts. The image of the mind looking out on the external world is actually a heroic image or heroic myth, in that it portrays the inner essence of the person existing in a state that is disconnected from all that sustains life. This myth, pervasive in the culture of Western industrial societies, we (Stolorow and Atwood, 1992) have termed the *myth of the isolated mind* (p. 7). It appears in many guises and variations. One can discern its presence in tales of invincible persons who overcome great adversity through solitary heroic acts, in philosophical works that revolve around a conception of an isolated, monadic subject, and in psychological and psychoanalytic doctrines that focus exclusively on processes occurring within the individual person. The latter includes, for example, Freud's vision of the mind as an impersonal machine that processes endogenous drive energies, ego psychology's autonomously self-regulating ego, and Kohut's pristine self with its preprogrammed inner design. We (Stolorow and Atwood, 1992) have argued that the pervasive, reified image of the mind in isolation, in all its many guises, is a form of defensive grandiosity that serves to disavow [human] vulnerability [and] embeddedness. . . . (pp. 41–42)

The consequences of isolated-mind thinking for psychoanalytic work are extensive and profound. Patients who meet an isolated-mind clinician may find themselves viewed as perfectionistic, narcissistic, or even borderline. Indeed, patients who have experience with isolated-mind mental health professionals may initially describe themselves to us similarly: "I am a borderline," "I am a manic-depressive," and so on. Later, we come to hear the experiential sense of what has been obliterated (compounding earlier invalidation) by these formulas: "I feel that I'm not real," "I feel I'm not inside my body," and so on. Within the psychoanalytic situation, patients are said to be projecting, identifying, resisting, or acting out. Such designations, almost always pejorative toward the patient, betray the clinician's continuing allegiance to the Cartesian mind and probably serve to protect us as therapists from our awareness of how we are ourselves implicated in what we too easily describe as "the patient's pathology." The atomism of isolated-mind thinking implies that people are not essentially related to each other, that their being is fundamentally self-enclosed. This self-enclosure also involves an ideal of self-sufficiency that Descartes himself described and advocated, as was discussed in the previous chapter.

A second prominent feature of Cartesian-mind thinking is the infamous subject-object split. Cartesian ontology claims that the object is real (existing independently of any knower) but that the subject *(cogito ergo sum)* is even more fundamentally real because self-evidently known. Whether or not one accepts Descartes's epistemological derivation of the external world from the isolated mind, with the innate idea of God as ultimate guarantor, the ontological division between mental and extended/physical realities has persisted in modern thought. Idealism took many forms: the immaterialism of Berkeley's *esse est percipi* (to be is to be perceived), the transcendental idealism of Kant, and the absolute idealism of Fichte and Hegel. In each of these views only the mental was fully or primordially real. On the other side, empiricists like Locke, Hume, and Mill claimed that mind was illusory or at best derivative. In twentieth-century psychology this view was taken to the extreme, eventuating in behaviorism; among philosophers it is often known as "eliminative materialism," wherein what is "eliminated" in the picture of human life is everything except its physical aspects. The whole dispute, however, depends on a full acceptance of the Cartesian premise of the subject-object split. This ontological chasm in turn enabled Locke to found modern epistemology on the notion of the idea or representation as the bridge between mind/subject and thing/object.

In psychoanalysis, this split appears in the contrast between psychical reality and external reality. Although Freud wanted to construct a model of the mind fully as mechanistic as the theories studied in physics and chemistry, his dependence on the biological theory of instinct gave psychical reality some organicity and flexibility. A variability was associated with the object of the subject's drives, as well as with their aims. Today, perhaps the residues of subject-object thinking persist most clearly in interpersonal theories, where a therapeutic relationship becomes described as an "interaction," and the "interaction" is analyzed in terms of the causal effects that people, understood though usually not acknowledged as essentially separate monads, are having on each other. Some object relations theories—the term gives the presuppositions away—speak unapologetically of the subject's objects, usually understood as mental contents. These mental contents fuse Descartes's objects with Locke's ideas and representations. Ironically, even theories of subject-subject relating may preserve the conception of subjectivity derived from the contrast between subject and object, that is, a Cartesian subject with all the features we are describing.

A third, almost universal feature of the Cartesian mind is the contrast between inner and outer. Inner reality is psychic; outer reality is material or extended in space. Again, the inner is subjective; the outer is objective, real, or external, depending on context. The mind is a container with ideas, fantasies, emotions, and even drives and instincts inside. External reality may affect this container and its contents, but it is always *external* reality. For Descartes himself, as noted in the previous chapter, this feature of mind served a powerful protective function, shielding the disengaged interiority from engagement with a dangerous outside. In psychoanalysis, ego psychology was built on the inner-outer contrast: psychological health meant the adaptation of the ego (Freud's *Ich*, though less substantialized than "the ego" sounds, was still inner) to the external world. Cavell (1993), drawing on the work of Wittgenstein and other philosophers, has extensively presented the philosophical criticisms of this inner-outer dichotomy and has explored its implications for psychoanalytic theory.

Practically speaking, this dichotomy is particularly dangerous in clinical work (Orange, 2002b). Patients and analysts can become endlessly entangled in trying to determine where a particular reality lies, inside or outside, or where responsibility for a reaction, for a life pattern, or for some interpersonal disaster lies. Tempted to think that everything is either inside or outside, and that these are genuine logical opposites, psychoanalytic theorists have described the Cartesian mind with spatial and mechanistic metaphors like transferring, displacing, and projecting, or have talked of distortion and delusion. Such conceptions may interfere with a shared search for profound and personal experiences of trauma, of self-loss, and of nonbeing (see Chapter 8).

Fourth, the Cartesian mind craves clarity and distinctness. The chaos, process, soft assembling, and emergence so dear to the systems thinking of the late twentieth century would turn poor Descartes over in his grave. Binary logic (true/false) proved robust and fruitful in the development of modern science, as Descartes's contemporary, Galileo, who read nature by cleaning out misleading sense experience, showed. But binary logic, with its best friend Occam's razor (the principle of parsimony), has demonstrated serious limitations even within its own spheres of applicability. It requires blindness to everything that does not fit, especially singularity and uniqueness. Even the computer, binary logic's creation, has required new and more "fuzzy" logics in order to more adequately address the nature of complex systems.[1]

The need for Cartesian clear and distinct ideas often appears in psychology as reductionism, the "it all comes down to" approach. Ironically, reductionism is easiest to see in the theories of others. As psychoanalysts, we see this

---

[1] Even these fuzzy logics are of course reducible to binary codes and therefore will never fully encompass the realms of subjective meaning that are the concern of the *Geisteswissenschaften* (human sciences). At the same time, we may question whether Dilthey's ([1883] 1989) famous distinction between the *Naturwissenschaften* and the *Geisteswissenschaften* may not contain its own residual Cartesian dualism. It does, however, remind us that subjective experience is not simply reducible to its material conditions. Nor, similarly, and this was Dilthey's concern, is understanding reducible to mere translation. Dilthey, like Husserl, both perpetuated and undermined Cartesian thinking.

clearly in behaviorism. Post-Freudians can see it in instinct theory. But do we also see the reductionism in our own favorites: selfobject theories, attachment theories, affect or trauma theories, or whatever the current fashion may be? Only a contrite "fallibilism"—Charles Sanders Peirce's word for a questioning attitude toward our own theories and formulations—and a devotion to dialogue with the possessors of other perspectives can help us to "make our ideas clear" (Peirce, 1878) without falling into the Cartesian search for simplicity that leads to reductionism.

In psychoanalysis, we can see that the search for certainty with its "clear and distinct ideas" criterion has both protected us from anxiety and restricted our creativity. Although psychoanalytic thinkers have always recognized complexity—overdetermination and multiple function are good examples of conceptualizing complexity—the search for clear and distinct ideas has persisted in procedural rules of "technique" (Orange, Atwood, and Stolorow, 1997) and in discussions of analyzability and correct interpretation. Aptly, the philosopher Richard Bernstein (1983) has called the concern for ultimate and certain foundations a kind of "Cartesian anxiety."

As a remedy for the Cartesian search for certainty, we have proposed, following American philosopher Peirce, the spirit of fallibilism (Orange, 2002a). This attitude includes both a continuing acknowledgment that we may at any time be mistaken and the understanding that truth can be sought only in a community of scholars, not by the philosophical or psychoanalytic lonesome cowboy. Additionally, we suggest the spirit of hermeneutics, which recommends taking any strange-sounding utterance as true, then seeking to understand how a reasonable person could think in this way. Only so can we begin a dialogue with what seems to us strange. We see both hermeneutics and fallibilism as powerful antidotes to Cartesian thinking, as did their more famous proponents, Hans-Georg Gadamer and Peirce. Now we would also suggest thinking more contextually and in terms of systems, but that can wait for the second part of this discussion.

A fifth feature of Cartesian thinking is its reliance on deductive logic. We might even call this "the Cartesian faith." There is no room for emotion, for art, or for the emergence of new *Gestalten* in the Cartesian mind. Freud, in this respect, deserves the revolutionary stature he claimed. He saw that such a mind must be exclusively conscious and thus could not account for psychological experience in health or illness, nor could it account for the rich productions of human culture with which he found himself surrounded in turn-of-the-century Vienna. Freud's solution, however, was to give the Cartesian house a basement where the genuine sources of psychic life lived. Unfortunately, the Freudian unconscious is equally isolated and atomistic, mechanistic, inner, and subjective as the Cartesian mind. It is simply hidden from view and imagined as operating according to its own internal logic (the primary process). Recently, however, several theorists (Bleichmar, 1999; Zeddies, 2000; Stolorow and Atwood, 1992) have attempted to describe and reconceptualize relational, intersubjectively generated forms of unconsciousness (see Chapter 3).

The absence of temporality is a sixth important feature of Cartesian thinking. It results, sooner or later, in what Taylor (1989) has called the "punctual self," the idea of an individual isolated as a point in space from other human beings and from the natural world. Worst of all, such a point in space is atemporal and thus has no developmental history, no story to tell. In psychoanalysis, the concept of transference both manifests and challenges the atemporal Cartesian mind. Past penetrates and shapes the experience of the present almost like a template, and past experience is always understood and reinterpreted *nachträglich*, in the light of what comes later. We do not use this Freudian word to suggest the unreality of what is so understood but rather to point to the continuing organization and reorganization of all experience. Indeed, Alfred Margulies (2000) has recently suggested that *Nachträglichkeit* is a relational process, an intersubjective phenomenon. At the same time, there is no doubt for Freudians, for object relations theorists who speak of old and new objects, and even for some proponents of systems theories that time is linear and one-dimensional. Old is old, and new is new, and the future usually drops out of consideration. (However, a good exception to this generalization can be found in the work of James Fosshage [1989] on the leading edge of dreams.) Clinically, we think this leads to some form of maturity morality— Kohut spoke of "reality-principle morality" (1984, p. 84) and of "a value-laden demand for psychological independence" (1991, p. 573)—in which we enjoin ourselves or our patients to grow up. "New" and "old" language can obscure the complexity, sometimes even the richness, of temporal experience and leave us wondering why our patients' experience, or our own, does not change in the ways we think it should.

Next, let us look at the furniture of the Cartesian mind: the ideas. For Descartes, and even more for his empiricist successors, ideas were copies or representations of things, conceived as individual items in the "external" world or as sense perceptions. Truth consisted of the correspondence of mental representations to external objects. This representational theory of mental contents persists in psychoanalysis to this day, among Freudians, for example, for whom dream images are representations of day residues fused with unconscious drive wishes. For object relations theorists, the mind is furnished with internal objects, and even among contemporary psychoanalysts influenced by infant research we find many forms of representation, often called schemata, or models. Indeed, for many of us, the still-Cartesian "representational world" of Joseph Sandler and Bernard Rosenblatt (1962) fortunately provided a stepping-stone and an impetus to move beyond Cartesian representational thinking into thinking about the psychological or experiential world (Stolorow, Atwood, and Ross, 1978; Atwood and Stolorow, 1980).

Clinically, the pernicious effects of representationalist thinking can be subtle. If, with our patients, we picture the mind as full of mental copies or representations, we can become much too concerned with the accuracy or inaccuracy of the copies and lose sight of the processes of creating and recreating meaning, of organizing and reorganizing experience. Any one of us may become mired in discussions with patients about what *really* happened, in the past or with us (see Chapter 6). We can also lose the forest for the trees, seeing images, ideas, memories, and fantasies as separate items in a mental file instead of attempting to understand with our patients the significance of whatever comes up for the sense of a whole life, a life in its rich or horrible contextuality.

Finally, but not last in importance, is the Cartesian concept of mind as substance. The mind, although stripped of corporeality and contrasted with extended substance (body), remains a thing, a thing that has an inside and that causally interacts with other things, for example, the body. Thus, the Cartesian substance is reified, made excessively abstract, and completely reduced to a commodity. "A mind is a terrible *thing* to waste." Psychoanalysis, misled by languages that tempt us to treat grammatical nouns as substantives (Wittgenstein, 1953), has reified psychological experience into mental contents like drives, fantasies, affects, and the like. This reduction of mind to thing, item, or substance can lead to underestimating the processes of human life that are genuinely mental: emoting, thinking, valuing, fantasizing, desiring, aesthetic experiencing, creating, and so on. Instead we revert to mechanistic metaphors of projecting, repressing, and transferring, that is, moving the mental contents around. Relinquishing these mechanistic and content-oriented metaphors can allow psychoanalysts of all persuasions more room to focus on experiential and systemic process (Orange, 2002c).

Experiential Worlds

World is perhaps the pivotal and defining concept of intersubjectivity theory, that is, of our systems view of psychoanalysis. We speak of subjective worlds, of worlds of experience, of personal universes. Psychoanalysis "is pictured here as a science of the intersubjective, focused on the interplay between the differently organized subjective worlds of the observer and the observed" (Atwood and Stolorow, 1984, p. 41). Or again, "the specific unfolding developmental needs of a particular child . . . are assimilated by the psychological world of each caretaker" (p. 68). An intersubjective field, the central theoretical construct of intersubjectivity theory, is defined as "a system composed of differently organized, interacting subjective worlds" (Stolorow, Brandchaft, and Atwood, 1987, p. ix). To distinguish this intersubjectivity theory from other uses of the term *intersubjective*, we have explained that "we use 'intersubjective' to refer to any psychological field formed by interacting worlds of experience, at whatever developmental level these worlds may be organized" (Stolorow and Atwood, 1992, p. 3). And again, "the concept of an intersubjective system brings to focus both the individual's world of [personal] experience and its embeddedness with other such worlds in a continual flow of reciprocal mutual influence" (p. 18). Similarly, attempting to situate intersubjectivity theory in a psychoanalytic historical context, one of us claimed that "the intersubjective approach shares the generality of scientific inquiry and the particularity of empathic concentration on one individual's organized and organizing subjective world" (Orange, 1995, p. 13). Maxwell Sucharov (1994), too, has explored the concept of world as living system. All of the collaborators of intersubjective systems theory have continued to work toward a fundamental and far-reaching shift in the concept of the human, from isolated minds and punctual selves (Taylor, 1989) toward a system-embedded, context-conscious sense of experiential worlds (Orange, Atwood, and Stolorow, 1997).

In addition to the contributions of Heidegger ([1927] 1962) discussed in the previous chapter, philosophical sources for the concept of an experiential world include the *Lebenswelt* (lifeworld) of Edmund Husserl ([1936] 1970)—his final attempt to transcend his own Cartesian enterprise—and the *être-au-monde* (being-toward-the-world) of Maurice Merleau-Ponty ([1945] 1962). Our thinking about these conceptual possibilities has also been influenced by the work of Wittgenstein ([1921] 1961, 1953, 1958) on world, contexts of meaning, language games, and forms of life.

Now let us consider some features of an experiential world, considered as a radical conceptual alternative to the Cartesian mind. In contrast to the isolation and atomism of the focus on "the intrapsychic," most contemporary psychoanalytic schools emphasize relatedness, dialogue, and even systems theory. Lewis Aron (1996) has masterfully surveyed contemporary relational theories in psychoanalysis and detailed their rejection and replacement of one-person psychologies. Yet theorists now writing have Cartesian thinking in their bones—it has become Western common sense—and the most careful thinkers revert to it at times. Taylor's (1989) account makes it clear that this development was not inevitable, that it was and continues to be possible to think otherwise. The current talk of dyads, particularly indebted to the detailed and painstaking studies of infant researchers, is in our view a significant beginning, but it does not go far enough toward understanding development or psychoanalysis in context. Thinking systemically requires that personal experience be understood as world (Heidegger, [1927] 1962), not just as interaction. The very concept of interaction needs redefinition as only one aspect of the development of emerging, organizing, and reorganizing psychological worlds. A child in treatment, for example, is embedded in relational worlds of home, treatment, school, and other environments and can in no adequate way be understood in exclusively dyadic terms (Gotthold, personal communication). A psychological or experiential world is relationally complex, chaotic, systemic, and emergent (Thelen, 1989).

In contrast to the subject-object assumption embedded in Cartesian thinking, the concept of an experiential world is perspectival, recognizing that "the only truth or reality to which psychoanalysis provides access is the subjective organization of experience understood in an intersubjective context" (Orange, 1995, p. 62), only one perspective on a larger reality. (See Chapter 6 for a detailed discussion of our concept of perspectival realism and its clinical implications.)

In contrast to the inner-outer division underpinning the Cartesian mind, the concept of a psychological world envisions a kind of double inhabiting. Compatible with gestalt psychology's figure and ground, dependent on the organizing activity of the viewer, and indebted to Wittgenstein's image of the world as the visual field in which the Cartesian subject does not exist, this experiential world replaces the Cartesian subject. A knower cannot be an item in the world. Instead, the experiential world seems to be both inhabited by and inhabiting of the human being. People live in worlds, and worlds in people. People live in their worlds of family, layers of culture and history, language, and taken-for-granted routines and responses (Schutz, 1970). In the words of Alfred Schutz, "My lifeworld is open to both past and future, in respect of my experiencing this world as having existed before my birth and as going to continue after my death" (pp. 135–136). At the same time, the world that one is inhabits one: one is the organized and organizing gestalt of experience that is a world, and one is never away from it, never an isolated mind. Descartes himself could think only in the languages that inhabited him and that were spoken in the worlds he inhabited. His meditations, the ultimate symbol of thinking in isolation, are in fact an invitation to his readers to think with him, to ask questions, and to be questioned by him. Perhaps all linguistic expression is evidence that the isolated mind, or "the self," is impossible, that world is the nature and condition for the possibility of individual human beings (Heidegger, [1927] 1962).

Clinically, such a focus on the experiential world inhabiting and being inhabited by a patient will surely encourage analysts' awareness of their participation in the process, but not to the exclusion of all other considerations. Recognizing the insufficiency of moving from isolated mind to isolated dyad, analysts will not continue to impute defenses like projective identification to their patients or to themselves, understanding these concepts as residues of Cartesian thinking (see Chapter 5). The human being cannot be reduced to a particular[2] case of a diagnosis, nor human experience to a particular case of a

---

[2] Individuality does not necessarily mean isolation. Nor does it mean reduction to instantiation of a generality (for example, diagnosis): "I distinguish radically between singularity *(Einzelheit)* or individuality on the one hand, and particularity *(Besonderheit)* on the other. I term individual what exists without an inner double, is beyond comparison, and cannot identically recur . . . In contrast, the particular is the specification of a universal (of a rule). It can be attained effortlessly by means of deduction. The particular relates to the general as the case to the rule. A case could never modify a rule. It can only instantiate or not instantiate a rule" (Frank, 1992, p. 15).

so-called mechanism of defense. Instead, defense can be understood as a relatively stable property of a system—organismic, intersubjective, or cultural—necessary to maintain psychological organization.

Perhaps the most striking shift comes in the rejection of "clear and distinct ideas" in favor of the complexity, nonlinearity, more-or-less quality, and general fallibilism of systems thinking. The experiential world can only fleetingly be the linear world of logic and reason for which Descartes and many since have longed. Analysts' security will come instead from the sense that they can rely on their emotional contexts enough to tolerate and explore with curiosity the endlessly open questions. Such a capacity in the clinician must surely reassure the patient more than any clear and distinct answers evoking their inevitable "Yes, but . . . " responses, indicating that we have reduced experience to a formula. The tendency to open rather than to foreclose conversation about meanings may be the most reliable marker of world-oriented psychoanalytic thinking, no matter what the clinician's original training.

Similarly, the concept of an experiential world can encompass a more-or-less sense of awareness, without the traditionally rigid boundaries between conscious and unconscious. Psychoanalysis will always, we suspect, be most interested in those aspects of experience least accessible to ordinary awareness. Still, analysts need not define their work as if they had a special esoteric knowledge of a language unknown to the uninitiated and could thus exclude people for being "not psychoanalytically trained" or ideas for being just "unpsychoanalytic." Psychoanalysts are trained to increase, not to create, attunement to the emotional, aesthetic, organized, more-or-less conscious aspects of experiential worlds, so that within a specific relational context these worlds can come to feel more understandable and flexible to those who inhabit and are inhabited by them.

In contrast to the "punctual self," or Cartesian subject, the experiential world is profoundly historical, temporal, and emergent. Psychological time, something for which clocks and calendars do not provide good metaphors, is enormously complex, and within it past, present, and future are not easily distinguishable. Biological systems may provide a better analogy. There is a plant in Crete that grows like a cactus for twenty years, flowers once (spectacularly), and dies that year. Its development, like ours, at all times includes its past, present, and future, including its death and the birth of future generations. Similarly, as psychoanalysis replaces the Cartesian self with the experiential world, it will become more and more interested in development, understood in terms of great temporal complexity ("nonlinear systems"). The cultural/historical worlds we inhabit and that inhabit us will also become of greater interest to psychoanalytic thinking.

Next, the representationalism of Cartesian thinking gives way to a dialogic (not dyadic), participatory, perspectival, and hermeneutic concept of understanding. To understand a person, we cannot enter that person's mind, catalog its mental furniture (ideas, affects, and fantasies), and write a case report. Rather, in the only conception of "empathic immersion" that makes sense in post-Cartesian thinking, the participants in the conversation (two or more) immerse themselves in the interplay of personal worlds of experience. Instead of asking ourselves as clinicians, "What is wrong with this person?" or "What misrepresentations reside in this person's mind?" we may ask, "What could be the aspects of a person's experiential world that would lead her to believe or feel that she is a murderer?" "What is the personal lifeworld like of someone who sits or lies on my couch and says he is not really in the room?" "What can a person who feels in this way expect or hope for?" Such questioning attitudes, possible within most psychoanalytic communities, assume that what the other says is comprehensible and that the task is understanding, not evaluation, classification, or judgment. This change of focus forms an important part of the "cash value," or practical clinical import, of replacing the Cartesian mind with the experiential world.

Finally, as we replace the Cartesian mind with the experiential world, mind as a thing, item, or substance gives way to mentality as a quality of organizing personal experience (including experiences of disorganization, disengagement, confusion, disintegration, and chaos). Talk of multiple selves, quite common in relational circles, gives way to variously organized experiential worlds, essentially relational but more or less actually related and more or less integrated. Personal experience is not mental substance; it is the lifeworld, complex in quality and temporality, "messy, fluid, and context-sensitive" (Thelen and Smith, 1994), of an organized and organizing living system.

3

World Horizons:
An Alternative to
the Freudian Unconscious

A mythology reflects its region.
—Wallace Stevens

The boundary is that from which something begins its presencing.
—Martin Heidegger

Sensibility does not simply record facts; it unfolds a world . . . from which they will not be able to escape.
—Emmanuel Levinas

Freud's "discovery" of the unconscious has been characterized as a second Copernican revolution in that it radically undermined the epistemological status of the self-conscious subject, which had been the centerpiece of Descartes's philosophy and of Enlightenment thought in general. From a Freudian perspective, Descartes's self-conscious *cogito* was exposed as a grandiose illusion; consciousness was shown to be a mere pawn of vast unconscious forces of which the subject was completely unaware. Nevertheless, the Freudian unconscious remained deeply saturated with the very Cartesianism to which it posed a challenge (Cavell, 1993). As we have noted, the Freudian unconscious and its contents are but a sealed-off, underground chamber within the Cartesian isolated mind.

Within the conversation of post-Cartesian, post-Freudian, relational psychoanalysis, what is left of "the unconscious"? Without the mechanistic and reductionistic thinking of Freudian metapsychology, we can no longer envision the dynamic unconscious as a subterranean locale from which derivatives of instinctual drives are pushing and pulling conscious experience. When we relegate the topographic model (Freud, [1900] 1953) of conscious, unconscious, and preconscious to the realm of metaphor —comparable in some ways to stories of heaven, hell, and purgatory, all with gatekeepers—we lose some of the evocative power of the Freudian unconscious. Similarly, when we see the structural theory (Freud, [1923] 1961a) of ego, id, and superego as elaborate and pernicious reification, completely untenable once we are committed to think phenomenologically about human psychology, have we anything left from Freud's second Copernican revolution?

Perhaps we do. We have the Freudian intuition, shared by all who have ever seen value in psychoanalysis, that human experience—including our own—involves "more than meets the eye," combined with the sense that whatever this "something more" may be, it is the key to what most profoundly ails us.

The Freudian Unconscious

Let us first consider the Freudian unconscious from Freud's point of view, so far as this is possible from ours today. In an ironic twist on the scientific empiricism dominant in the world from which Freud so much wanted acceptance, the unconscious, not at all open to verification or measurement, was for him the absolute measure of truth. He (Freud, [1915] 1957) even appealed to Kant for inspiration:

> The psycho-analytic assumption of unconscious mental activity . . . [is] an extension of the corrections undertaken by Kant of our views on external perception. Just as Kant warned us not to overlook the fact that our perceptions are subjectively conditioned and must not be regarded as identical with what is perceived though unknowable, so psycho-analysis warns us not to equate perceptions by means of consciousness with the unconscious mental processes which are their object. (p. 171)

Freud further used a Kantian, or transcendental, form of argument to justify his claim that mind is in itself unconscious. Consciousness, he believed, is full of holes. Not only do troubled people who come for psychoanalysis exhibit symptoms that are, at best, counterproductive and, at worst, create for their possessors a life of torture, but in addition, ordinary daily experience is full of forgetting, slips of the tongue, and other parapraxes. All of us have dreams that are hard to decipher. Most of all, thought Freud, there is repression, which creates many lacunae in conscious experience and makes our lives difficult to understand. Therefore, Freud argued, we must assume that the psychically "real" is unconscious and that consciousness is only an epiphenomenon. The unconscious, by definition something that could not be directly experienced, was the result of an inference. It must exist, or we could not see the connections in our lives. It provides the missing links.

We now consider some features of the Freudian unconscious. It is, above all, the source of truth about human nature. Orthodox Freudians (along with Kleinians) hold a profoundly pessimistic view of human nature, according to which, in their version of original sin, we are by nature filled with incestuous lust and destructive rage. These live largely in the unconscious, unknown by the subject, who represses them whenever they or their derivatives erupt into consciousness but who nonetheless suffers from the distortions that repression creates in experience and living. Only an analyst, who possesses esoteric knowledge of the universal contents of this unconscious realm, can lead the way down into the patient's private hell, and thus back out into relief, or at least into a more conscious acceptance of the required renunciations. Or, in a Freudian metaphor for the detached expert, the patient needs a psychological surgeon who skillfully penetrates and rearranges the unconscious insides of the patient. The Freudian concept of the unconscious, with contents dictated by theoretical doctrine and already "known" by the analyst prior to any collaborative exploration, is responsible for many of the authoritarian features of traditional analysis. With privileged knowledge of the unconscious, the analyst is readily viewed as a *Besserwisser*, or "know-it-all." The analyst possesses truth, the patient only distortions and unawareness.

The Freudian unconscious functions as a reified and substantialized storehouse for whatever the conscious subject cannot tolerate. Whether, as one Freudian metaphor would have it, we envision the unconscious as a seething cauldron of incestuous and aggressive instinctual desires or as just a somewhat disorderly mental museum, this unconscious mind is a container. Granted, it contains more than a Cartesian *cogito*, and surely its contents are neither clear nor distinct. It also contains more than Lockean ideas, though these are surely there in the form of representations or mental copies of lived experiences. The Freudian unconscious contains mental pictures and drive derivatives such as wishes, impulses, and affects, all related, Freud believed, in lawful ways. Most important, the unconscious contains all that has been repressed.

The concept of repression cannot be separated from the Freudian unconscious. What is unconscious has been repressed, or will be if it ever slips into conscious awareness, and what is repressed automatically enters and lives in the unconscious. In Freud's early work, one's becoming conscious of the repressed causes unpleasure; in his later work, such awareness evokes psychic conflict. There is always much to hide: originally, the drive derivatives themselves; and later, all the compromises we have made to keep them out of awareness. Both repression and the unconscious are inherent in the Freudian view of human nature, which includes a basic sense of one's native badness and shamefulness. Familial and other developmental contexts are peripheral to the whole story of the Freudian unconscious, in that the child and his or her infantile instinctual wishes are the fundamental source of later problems. The unconscious is thus pictured as the home and source of innate, ahistorical, decontextualized evil.

While heavily steeped in Cartesian isolated-mind thinking, this vision of the unconscious can also be seen to have served powerful psychological functions for Freud. In our (Atwood and Stolorow, 1993) psychobiographical study of the personal, subjective origins of Freud's metapsychology, we found that Freud protected himself from awareness of the profound emotional impact of a series of early painful disappointments and betrayals by his mother by attributing his sufferings to his own omnipotent inner badness—that is, his incestuous lust and murderous hostility—a defensive translocation that found its way into his important adult relationships, including those with Wilhelm Fliess and with his wife, as well as into his formulations of clinical cases. Freud also imported this defensive solution, a form of defensive grandiosity, into his theory of psychosexual development and pathogenesis, a theory in which the primary pathogens were believed to be the unruly instinctual drives buried deep within the unconscious interior of the psyche. In this theoretical vision, idealized images of the parents, especially the mother, were preserved, allowing Freud ([1933] 1964), in a remarkable statement, to characterize the relationship between a mother and her son as "altogether the most perfect, the most free from ambivalence of all human relationships" (p. 133), and to apply the Oedipus myth in a manner that completely neglected the central role of the father's filicidal urge in setting the tragic course of events in motion. This same defensive principle fatefully shaped Freud's view of the psychoanalytic situation, wherein the cordon sanitaire that he wrapped around the parents he also wrapped around the presumptively neutral analyst, so that the patient's transference experiences could be seen as arising solely from unconscious contents within the isolated mind of the patient rather than being codetermined by the impact and meanings of the stance and activities of the analyst.

An Alternative: World Horizons

Let us now bring a set of assumptions different from Freud's to the problem of unconsciousness in human psychological life. We begin not with a Cartesian isolated mind-entity equipped with conscious, preconscious, and unconscious compartments, but with the concept of a multiply contextualized experiential world—a cornerstone of our intersubjective perspective. In place of Freud's topographical and structural theories of mind, we envision an organized totality of lived personal experience, more or less conscious and more or less contoured according to those emotional convictions or organizing principles formed in a lifetime of emotional and relational experiences. Instead of a container, we picture an experiential system of expectations, interpretive patterns, and meanings, especially those formed in the contexts of psychological trauma—losses, deprivations, shocks, injuries, violations, and the like. Because such convictions and ordering principles usually operate outside the domain of reflective self-awareness, we have characterized them as prereflectively unconscious (Atwood and Stolorow, 1980, 1984). Within such a system or world, one can feel and know certain things, often repetitively and with unshakable certainty. Whatever a person is not able to feel or know falls outside the horizons (Gadamer, [1975] 1991) of his or her experiential world, requiring no container. The rigidity associated with various kinds of psychopathology can be grasped as a kind of freezing of a person's experiential horizons so that other perspectives remain unavailable. Or we could say that a person is always organizing his or her emotional and relational experiences so as to exclude whatever feels unacceptable, intolerable, or too dangerous in particular intersubjective contexts.

Psychoanalysis, in this view, is no longer an archaeological excavation of ever deeper layers of an isolated and substantialized unconscious mind. Instead, it is a dialogic exploration of a patient's experiential world, conducted with awareness of the unavertable contribution of the analyst's experiential world to the ongoing exploration. Such empathic-introspective inquiry seeks understanding of what the patient's world feels like, of what emotional and relational experiences it includes, often relentlessly, and what it assiduously excludes and precludes. It seeks comprehension of the network of convictions, the rules or principles that prereflectively organize the patient's world and keep the patient's experiencing confined to its frozen horizons and limiting perspectives. By illuminating such principles in a dialogic process and by grasping their life-historical origins, psychoanalysis aims to expand the patient's experiential horizons, thereby opening up the possibility of an enriched, more complex, and more flexible emotional life.

We turn now to some further theoretical and clinical implications of our conception of unconsciousness in terms of the limiting horizons of an experiential world. First and foremost, unlike the repression barrier, which Freud viewed as a fixed intrapsychic structure within an isolated mind, world horizons, like the experiential worlds they delimit, are conceptualized as emergent properties of ongoing dynamic, relational systems (Stolorow, 1997). Forming and evolving within a nexus of living systems, experiential worlds and their horizons are recognized as being exquisitely context-sensitive and context-dependent. The horizons of awareness are thus fluid and ever-shifting, products both of the person's unique intersubjective history and of what is or is not allowed to be known within the intersubjective fields that constitute his or her current living. Our conception of world horizons as emergent features of intersubjective systems bears a kinship to Samuel Gerson's (1995) and Timothy Zeddies's (2000) idea of a "relational unconscious" and Donnel Stern's (1997) discussion of "unformulated experience." Stern, whose views, like our own, have been strongly influenced by Gadamer's philosophical hermeneutics, has claimed as we do that it is the relational field that "structures the possibilities of knowing—the potential for what we can say and think and what we cannot" (p. 31).

Our ideas about world horizons have developed over the course of more than two decades from our attempts to describe the intersubjective origins of differing forms of unconsciousness (Atwood and Stolorow, 1980, 1984; Stolorow and Atwood, 1989, 1992). Our evolving theory rested on the assumption that the child's conscious experience becomes progressively articulated through the validating attunement of the early surround (see also Coburn, 2001). Two closely interrelated but conceptually distinguishable forms of unconsciousness were pictured as developing from situations of massive malattunement. When a child's experiences are consistently not responded to or are actively rejected, the child perceives that aspects of his or her own experience are unwelcome or damaging to the caregiver. These regions of the child's experiential world must then be sacrificed in order to safeguard the needed tie. Repression was grasped here as a kind of negative organizing principle, always embedded in ongoing intersubjective contexts, determining which configurations of conscious experience were not to be allowed to come into full being. In addition, we argued, other features of the child's experience may remain unconscious, not because they have been repressed but because, in the absence of a validating intersubjective context, they simply were never able to become articulated. This form of unconsciousness would seem to be closely similar to Donnel Stern's (1997) concept of unformulated experience— uninterpreted "material that has never been *brought into* consciousness" (p. xii, emphasis in original). With both forms of unconsciousness, the horizons of awareness were pictured as taking form in the medium of the differing responsiveness of the surround to different regions of the child's experience. This conceptualization was seen to apply to the psychoanalytic situation as well, wherein the patient's "resistance" can be shown to fluctuate in concert with perceptions of the analyst's varying receptivity and attunement to the patient's experience.

During the preverbal period of infancy, the articulation of the child's experience is achieved through attunements communicated in the sensorimotor dialogue with caregivers. With the maturation of the child's symbolic capacities, symbols gradually assume a place of importance alongside sensorimotor attunements as vehicles through which the child's experience is validated within the developmental system. Therefore, we argued, in that realm of experience in which consciousness increasingly becomes articulated in symbols, unconscious becomes coextensive with unsymbolized. When the act of articulating an experience is perceived to threaten an indispensable tie, repression can now be achieved by preventing the continuation of the process of encoding that experience in symbols.

Interestingly, the foregoing description of repression bears a close similarity to Donnel Stern's (1997) view of dissociation, which he has defined as a "refusal to interpret" (p. xii) experience, a defensive "avoidance of verbal [symbolic] articulation" (p. 114). He, in turn, equated dissociation with unformulated experience. We think it would be better to speak here of *dysformulated* experience, thereby distinguishing the active aborting of a symbolizing process believed to be too dangerous from a situation wherein a symbolizing process did not occur in the first place.

What seems particularly interesting, though, is that whereas historically psychoanalysts have attempted to distinguish sharply between repression and dissociation, Stern has used the word *dissociation* to designate virtually the same process—the aborting of symbolization—that we have called repression. What can this mean? We think it means that in a post-Cartesian philosophical world, with no subject-object bifurcation, no cognition-affect split, and no isolated unconscious mind-entities containing contents, it is no longer so necessary or compelling to make the sharp distinctions implied in such terms as repression, dissociation, splitting, denial, and disavowal. From a contextualist viewpoint, we can recognize such terms as referring to all the varieties of limiting world horizons, of disclosure and hiddenness, which reflect patterns of organizing activity formed and maintained within living, intersubjective systems.

A Case of Unconsciousness Revisited

To illustrate our view of unconsciousness in terms of contextualized experiential worlds and their limiting horizons, we revisit a dramatic instance of unconsciousness illuminated during an analysis conducted nearly thirty years ago by one of us while he was a candidate in training (Stolorow, 1974). At the time of the treatment, the case was formulated according to the assumptions of Freudian ego psychology, which included the characteristics of the Freudian unconscious that we described earlier. Here we first present an abridged summary of the case as it was understood then, excerpted from a published report (Stolorow and Lachmann, 1975). Then we will take another look from an intersubjective systems perspective.

When Anna began her four-year analysis, she was thirty-one years old. She had been married for twelve years and worked as an executive. She complained of both diffuse anxiety and states of acute panic, the content of which centered around fantasies that her husband would leave her for another woman.

Anna was born in Budapest, where, in her early years, she lived through the horrors of World War II and the Nazi occupation. When she was four years old, her father was taken to a concentration camp, where he eventually died. During an analytic session, while exploring the ways in which she kept aspects of her relationship with her father alive in her current experiences with men, Anna made a startling discovery that proved to be pivotal in her treatment. She suddenly realized that she had never accepted the reality of her father's death. Indeed, she exclaimed that she believed even now with a feeling of *absolute conviction* that her father is still alive. Much of the remainder of her analysis was concerned with uncovering the genetic roots and characterological consequences of this firmly embedded conviction.

At age four, Anna had not yet developed the cognitive capacities that would have enabled her on her own to comprehend the meaning of the terrible events that were taking place around her, especially the sudden and inexplicable disappearance of her father. The surviving adults in Anna's environment, particularly her mother, failed to provide sufficient assistance to her in the task of integrating the grim realities of the war and her father's incarceration and death. The mother falsified the reality of the war, telling Anna that the exploding bombs were just doors slamming. She also pretended to Anna that the father had not been taken to a concentration camp and tacitly perpetuated the myth that he was alive by never directly discussing his death with Anna and never openly mourning his loss. These experiences left Anna with a feeling of confusion about what was real and what was unreal, a feeling that was reactivated in her analysis with the discovery of her unconscious conviction that her father was still alive. It was left to Anna's own fantasy life to fill the vacuum left by maternal omissions and falsifications in order to make some sense of these incomprehensible and tragic events and regain some feeling of mastery:

"I had to find some reason. It all seemed so crazy. I couldn't accept that such things could happen and there was nothing you could do. I was trying to understand what was happening. None of the adults would tell me. No one sat down with me and told me my father was in a concentration camp or dead. So I made up my own explanations."

The specific content of the fantasies which Anna elaborated to "explain" her father's disappearance and continued absence developed as the complex consequence of several factors, including her level of ego development, the particular circumstances surrounding her father's disappearance, and her level of psychosexual development at the time of his loss.

With regard to ego development, there is evidence that a child at age four has not yet attained the abstract concept of death as a final and irreversible cessation of life. To the extent that a death is acknowledged at all, it is typically conceived of as a potentially reversible departure to a distant geographical location. A common element in all of the conscious fantasies with which Anna explained her father's absence was the notion that he was living somewhere in Russia and might someday return to her. Throughout her childhood and on into adulthood, at first consciously and later unconsciously, she "waited and waited" for him to come back to her and feared that she might "miscalculate" or "do something wrong" that would make her miss her "last chance" to see him.

Consistent with this level of ego and superego development, Anna in her fantasy explanations blamed herself for her father's departure and continued absence. The particular circumstances surrounding his departure contributed to the content of her fantasies. It was actually Anna herself who had found and brought to her father the notice instructing him to report to a concentration camp.

She did not understand what it was and so took it very lightly. She even felt excited about the opportunity to deliver something to her father. When she gave the notice to him, she danced around him in a very happy and excited mood. Later, she discovered that the notice meant her father would have to go away, and she felt she had done a terrible thing to him by being so happy. After he was gone, she developed a fantasy that he hated her for being happy when she delivered the notice because her happiness meant she did not care about him. She further fantasized that if only she had demonstrated her love and devotion by becoming "hysterical enough" about the notice, then he would have returned to her.

The final elements for Anna's fantasy explanations of her father's disappearance—perhaps the most fateful ones for her characterological development—were provided by the vicissitudes of her psychosexual development. Because her father had been taken away when she was four years old, Anna's explanations of his absence contained derivatives of both castration anxiety and the oedipal stage. She developed fantasies that her father stayed away because she was defective, repulsive, and totally valueless to him. And she developed further fantasies that he stayed away because he had met another woman in Russia and had chosen to stay there and live with her: If Anna could just win him away from the woman who had stolen him, he would return.

Material that unfolded in the course of her analysis suggested that castration derivatives played the more prominent role in her interpretation of her father's absence. The loss of her father intensified and "fixated" the feelings of narcissistic mortification characteristic of the castration anxiety phase, a time when Anna looked to her father for a feeling of wholeness and self-worth. The importance of castration anxiety in Anna's reaction to the loss of her father was supported by the important role that a clear-cut illusory penis played in her development. From her early childhood, Anna had maintained a fully conscious conviction that a small penis protruded from her vulva, a conviction which obviously held disastrous consequences for her developing self-image and sense of sexual identity.

It is questionable whether the various explanatory and restitutive fantasies discussed so far technically fall within the category of defensive denial fantasies. Primarily, they seem to represent attempts on the part of a four-year-old child to adapt to a state of cognitive insufficiency, that is, to fill in with phase-specific fantasy elaborations the cognitive vacuum left by an immature ego inadequately supported by the surviving adults in her environment.

At some point after the war, during her latency period when cognitive and ego maturation and expanded sources of information had enabled Anna to begin to register and comprehend the realities of her father's incarceration and death, she indeed began to construct an elaborate defensive denial-in-fantasy system that, until its dissolution by analysis, functioned to keep her father alive. Her efforts at this later point can properly be described as a denial that warded off the mourning process of which she was now becoming developmentally capable. The denial was promoted by the libidinal, the aggressive, and the self-preservative components of her complex, ambivalent attachment to him.

In constructing the denial-in-fantasy system, Anna made ample use of the ready-made fantasies by which she had originally explained her father's absence. In order to deny his death, she now had to cling to both the castration derivatives and fantasies of oedipal defeat. And to maintain this denial system, she had to select and cling to negative memories of her father's devaluing, rejecting, and excluding her—and repress all positive memories of his loving, caring for, and valuing her lest they contradict and jeopardize her denial fantasies. In her adult life, Anna further buttressed her denial system by clinging to real or imagined experiences in which a father surrogate devalued or rejected her or was devoted to another woman. This, in turn, reinforced her conviction that her father was rejecting of her or chose another woman but was still alive. Furthermore, she warded off experiences of feeling loved, valued, or chosen by a man so that her denial fantasies and her devotion and loyalty to her father would not be jeopardized.

It was between the age of ten and early adolescence that circumstances necessitated the final consolidation of Anna's denial fantasies into a static and unassailable system. When Anna was ten, her mother remarried, and Anna's denial fantasies dovetailed with a host of oedipal-competitive and sexual conflicts, greatly intensified and complicated by Anna's hope that her stepfather would substitute for her lost father. At this point, Anna, in reality a bright and pretty child, began to feel ugly, stupid, defective, and "freaky" and became obsessively preoccupied with her illusory penis—symptoms that remained with her until they were removed by the analysis.

The mother's remarriage represented to Anna the first tacit acknowledgment of her father's death by the adults in her environment. This threatened abruptly to obliterate her denial fantasies. Hence, Anna was forced to redouble her efforts at denial and restitution and to fortify all of the mechanisms by which she was keeping her father alive. Moreover, she had to mobilize feelings of being totally unloved and abused by her stepfather, because to recognize and accept his affection and caring would mean accepting that her father too had loved and valued her and was therefore absent because he was dead. By warding off the stepfather with various castration derivatives, Anna insured that she would not "miscalculate" by accepting her father's death and accepting her stepfather, and that she, unlike her mother, would be ready and waiting for her father when he returned.

The final consolidation of her denial system occurred during Anna's early adolescence as her pubertal development exacerbated the threat of overt sexual activity with her stepfather. In response to her stepfather's sexual intrusiveness and seductiveness, Anna would think to herself, "My real father would never do such things" and wistfully yearn for her real father's return. She elaborated fantasies in which he would return from Russia, her mother would choose to stay with the stepfather, and Anna would remain with her real father and enjoy his care and protection. This necessitated a final consolidation of the denial fantasies, through which she kept her father alive, into a static defensive system with all its unfortunate consequences for Anna's self-image, self-esteem, and patterns of relating to men.

Much of the above history was of course recapitulated in the transference. During the period when the analytic work consisted of active confrontations with the denial fantasies and encouragement for Anna to accept the reality of the father's death, she became immersed in rage-filled transference struggles in which she cast the analyst in the image of the sexually intrusive stepfather who threatened to destroy her devotion and loyalty to her real father.

The therapeutic alliance withstood the impact of these transference storms, and Anna was eventually able to work through the transference and give up her denial system. The most immediate consequence was that she experienced a belated mourning process as she permitted herself to imagine the horrors and prolonged, tortured death her father must have suffered at the hands of the Nazis. (At this point she also began to fear the analyst would die.) Coincident with this unfolding mourning process was Anna's dramatic recovery of positive memories of a loving father; along with these memories, she also retrieved repressed memories of loving devotion from various other men. Anna now clearly recognized that she had elaborated a complex denial system in which she viewed herself as defective and sacrificed her memories of her father's and other men's love in order to spare her father the terrible, agonizing death she now realized he must have experienced. Just as the sacrifices she endured to keep him alive were a measure of her great love for her father, so now was her pain in belatedly imagining how he died.

Predictably, as Anna accepted and mourned the death of her father, she also began to give up the feelings of being defective and undesirable. The working through of her denial system and her father's death had made possible the uncovering and reintegration of the repressed split-off image of the loving father. This in turn resulted in marked and lasting improvements in her self-image and self-esteem and in increasingly strong feelings of being valued and desired by men in her current life (Stolorow and Lachmann, 1975, pp. 600–609).

The foregoing case report demonstrates that the Freudian unconscious provides a coherent and compelling explanatory account of a dramatic instance of unconsciousness, so long as one leaves unchallenged the Cartesian isolated-mind assumptions that saturate Freudian theory. How is our understanding of the case altered if we rethink it from an intersubjective systems viewpoint? Can we thereby arrive at a more comprehensive theoretical explanation of the therapeutic process and its results?

For one thing, the psychosexual fantasies—that is, the recurring images of genital defectiveness and rivalrous defeat—that pervaded this analysis can no longer be viewed as manifestations of an innate, decontextualized, instinctual bedrock, a hard-wired epigenetic master plan presumed to predetermine the developmental trajectories of all human beings. Instead, we view such concrete imagery as dramatic symbolizations of the themes that came to dominate Anna's experiential world, themes that crystallized in the patterns of intersubjective transaction that took place between Anna and her caregivers over the course of her psychological development. These relational patterns and resulting principles of organization were, of course, themselves influenced by the historical, cultural, and linguistic contexts in which they were embedded.

Even Anna's so-called cognitive capacities at the time of her father's death, which contributed heavily to her interpretations of this tragic event, must be contextualized. What Anna could know of her father's death was codetermined by her sense of what her caregivers could and could not permit her to know. The "maternal omissions and falsifications" mentioned in the published case report were not simply a failure to assist Anna in the task of integrating the grim realities of the war and her father's death. They were also powerful messages to Anna concerning what perceptions and knowledge were not permissible and tolerable within the developmental system. Anna's "inability" to know her father's death and her later denial of it can be understood, in part, as compliance with her mother's requirement that she not know, a compliance that became tightly woven into the fabric of Anna's perceptual world, fixing the experiential horizons that so sharply limited her self-esteem and sense of herself in relationships with men.

A further contextualization of Anna's unconsciousness is achieved when we focus on her affectivity. As we stressed in the introductory chapter, the shift from drive to affect as the central motivational principle for psychoanalysis is one of the hallmarks of intersubjectivity theory. This shift is of great theoretical importance, we said, because it automatically entails a contextualization of both human motivation and unconsciousness. As Aron (1996) has noted, a focus on affect has been characteristic of much contemporary psychoanalytic theory. The contextualizing implications of such a focus were anticipated in Harry Stack Sullivan's (1953) discussion of the reciprocal contagion of anxiety that can occur between a mother and her child.

A prominent affect state pervading Anna's experiential world was omitted from the published case report even though it appeared abundantly in the clinical process notes—namely, what Anna called her "nameless terror." This affect state, which came to be grasped as over-

whelming feelings of aloneness, vulnerability, and help-
lessness in a dangerous, annihilating world, was frequently
revived in the analysis as she remembered and pictured the
horrors of the war years and Nazi occupation and, especially, her father's incarceration and death. For our purposes here, the most important characteristic of these
traumatized states is that the terror was "nameless." How
is this to be understood?

Clearly, the "maternal omissions and falsifications" discussed earlier not only curtailed Anna's knowing but had
a powerfully aborting impact on her affective development as well. She portrayed her mother as being oblivious
to Anna's emotional experience in general. Surely a
mother who needed to falsify the horrors occurring
around her family on a daily basis could not provide articulating, validating attunement to her daughter's terror
and other painful feelings. Hence, until articulated in
analysis, the most painful and frightening regions of
Anna's affectivity remained incompletely symbolized—
"nameless." Additionally, it seems likely that she experienced her mother's falsifications as an indication that
Anna's painful feelings were unwelcome, an injunction
not to feel or name her own affective pain, to keep her
most unbearable emotional states outside the horizons of
symbolized experience. Hence, yet another source—perhaps the most important—of the denial system that kept
her father alive was Anna's compliance with her mother's
requirement that she not feel or utter her own grief.

Let us now reconsider further Anna's psychosexual
fantasies from an experiential-world perspective. Anna's
world was shattered by a traumatic loss that could not be
assimilated, not only because it was surrounded by

unspeakable horror but also because no one acknowledged it. Her fantasies can be grasped as desperate attempts to reassemble an experiential world from the shards of disaster, in the face of her mother's lies. She needed to make sense of the glaring disparity between her own experience of loss and others' denial. This sense-making required ever more elaborate efforts to fill in the missing pieces of her traumatically destroyed life. Her fantasies are no longer seen as derivatives of unconscious instinctual drives but rather as a creative expression of the fundamental need to organize her experience. Given enough traumatic shock, which, as we have written, includes the contexts of denial, indifference, and invalidation, such fantasies can become rigid and, as seen with Anna, quite crippling. Yet no matter how bizarre they may appear to be, they can be understood as attempts to name what is nameless.

Finally, let us contextualize the gains that Anna achieved in her analysis by considering another crucial element left out of the published report: the analyst's transference relationship with his patient, which he explored in his own analysis. The analyst had loved his own mother dearly and, throughout his childhood and adolescence, had yearned to find ways to unlock the emotional aliveness he believed was encased behind the wall of her chronic wooden depression. These feelings were strongly revived in his relationship with Anna, for whom he cared deeply. Once Anna's denial of her father's death had been revealed, the analyst quickly saw her aborted grief as the key that could unlock her shackled affective vitality. If he could reach her grief, then he could do for Anna what he had never been able to do for his mother.

Unlike Anna's mother, who could not tolerate her daughter's grief, the analyst wanted and welcomed it, and this, we believe, was a powerfully therapeutic element that helped her give up the denial system and embrace a view of herself as a desired, valued, and loved woman.

The widening of Anna's experiential horizons that was taking place within the therapeutic relationship was concretized in a dramatic revision of her life history that occurred during the period in which she was letting go of the denial system and beginning to grieve for her father. She began a session by reminding the analyst of the "cruddy old yellow doll carriage" her father had given her that for so long had remained a symbol of her father's lack of love for her. Then she said she had remembered something she had "completely forgotten": that originally her father had bought her a "brand new, really beautiful" pink doll carriage. During the session, she remembered overhearing her family discussing a tricycle as a possible gift for her, but her father objected, insisting that a pretty little girl should have a beautiful doll carriage. She recalled further that one day she took her precious carriage to a playground and let another girl use it, that the latter walked away with it, and that it was never found again. Her father had bought the cruddy yellow carriage as a replacement for the one that had been lost. (The memory of the beautiful doll carriage being stolen and replaced by a cruddy *yellow* one may also have been a screen memory metaphorically encoding the devastating impact of Anna's experiences of anti-Semitic persecution.) She said she now understood that "forgetting" the first beautiful carriage, a symbol of her father's love, served the fantasies through which she kept him alive by "explaining" why he failed to return to her, and she soon remembered many other instances of her father's loving her. The recovery of the beautiful doll carriage also symbolized the process that was occurring in the relationship with her analyst, in whom she had found both a mother who could help her grieve and the lost loving father of her childhood. Like constricting world horizons, expanding horizons of awareness too can only be grasped in terms of the intersubjective contexts within which they take form.

Anna's analyst created with her a hospitable home for her nameless terror. His recognition of her need to grieve allowed her to know, to name, and to reorganize the horror of an early traumatic loss in which she had remained painfully trapped. This loss, outside the horizons of the world her mother could permit her, required the creative work of fantasy, but these fantasies became calcified because they remained insulated from dialogue and questioning. Such questioning dialogue is indispensable if a psychological world is to develop and expand. And it is this questioning dialogue, not the excavation of an isolated unconscious mind, that constitutes the quintessential work of psychoanalysis.

In reaction to our reconceptualization of Anna's analysis, colleagues have posed the question: How would this new understanding have altered the conduct of Anna's treatment? The conceptual shift with the clearest therapeutic implications concerns Anna's inability to know her father's death, which we now see less as a product of her limited cognitive capacities at the time of the loss and more as compliance with her mother's requirement that Anna's grief remain unnamed. Leaving aside the considerable difficulties involved in postdicting a change in the course of an analysis conducted thirty years ago, it seems to us that the different understanding of Anna's unconsciousness might have significantly altered the analytic approach to her "rage-filled transference struggles" during the period when her analyst actively confronted her denial fantasies and encouraged her to accept her father's death. With the aid of this new understanding, he might have inquired, repeatedly throughout the period of these struggles, whether Anna feared that he would be intolerant of her emerging grief as her mother had been, and whether she was responding to anything from him that lent itself to such an expectation. Was she thus experiencing his confrontations and encouragement as invitations to disaster for the therapeutic relationship? The illumination of this emotional conviction organizing Anna's experience of the analytic exchange might have significantly deepened the therapeutic bond and expanded even further her capacity to grieve and, more broadly, to experience, name, and integrate painful affect.

Upon further reflection, however, the foregoing hindsight must be tempered with the realization that at the time of the analysis, a change was already beginning to take place in the analyst's perspective. Anna's young analyst was already working contextually with her, even though his guiding framework, still in germinal form, was as yet unformulated, prereflective, nameless. It was only years later, when the communitarian context of *his* thinking could permit a widening of *his* world horizons, that this pretheoretical aspect of his developing clinical style could be articulated and named as an intersubjective systems perspective on pathogenesis and the therapeutic process. It is our belief that any such expansion of an analyst's theoretical horizons will have a salutary impact on therapeutic outcome, to the degree that such expansion enhances the analyst's capacity to grasp features of the patient's experiential world hitherto obscured. Yet, insofar as the analytic dyad functions as a complex, nonlinear, dynamic system (Stolorow, 1997), the specific therapeutic impact of change in any one of its elements (such as the analyst's theory) cannot be precisely forecasted. When we first began to develop our ideas about the role of the intersubjective context in the analytic process (Stolorow, Atwood, and Ross, 1978), we could not have predicted all of the ramifications of this enlarging perspective for therapeutic practice and effectiveness—in the treatment of psychotic states, for example (see Chapter 8). The attitude we bring to our theories of therapeutic action is thus a fallibilistic one (see Chapter 6), holding them lightly rather than tightly. Within the changing horizons of our current psychoanalytic world, much is yet unknown.

4

Kohut and Contextualism

The I makes its appearance ... through the world's being my world.
—**Ludwig Wittgenstein**

The world ... is the natural setting of, and field for, all my thoughts and all my explicit perceptions.... [M]an is in the world and only in the world does he know himself.
—**Maurice Merleau-Ponty**

The most that an original figure can hope to do is to recontextualize his or her predecessors. He or she cannot aspire to produce works that are themselves uncontextualizable.
—**Richard Rorty**

Our aim in this chapter is to paint a portrait of Heinz Kohut as a pivotal transitional figure in the development of a post-Cartesian, fully contextual psychoanalytic psychology. We discuss both his efforts to emancipate psychoanalytic theory from the tradition of Cartesian isolated-mind thinking and the extent to which his views remained caught within its very grip. Hence, as we honor

his great historical importance in the evolution of psychoanalytic thought, we will also pose a challenge to those
who regard his words as the first and the last.

Let us first approach our topic contextually, by examining one type of context—the historical. We begin with a
discussion of the historical origins and development of
Kohut's contextualism, and of our own.

The early germs of our psychoanalytic contextualism
can be found in a series of psychobiographical studies, conducted in the mid-1970s, in which we explored the personal, subjective origins of the theoretical systems of Freud,
Jung, Wilhelm Reich, and Otto Rank, studies that formed
the basis of our first book, *Faces in a Cloud* (Stolorow and
Atwood, 1979). Although the concept of *inter*subjectivity
was not introduced in the first edition of this book, it was
clearly implicit in the demonstrations of how the subjective
world of a psychological theorist profoundly influences his
or her understanding of other people's experiences. From
these studies we concluded that what psychoanalysis needs
is a theory of subjectivity itself—a unifying framework that
can account not only for the phenomena that other theories
address but also for these theories themselves. We were thus
led inexorably to a wholly phenomenological conception of
psychoanalysis. In our vision, psychoanalytic theory, at all
levels of abstraction and generality, was to be a depth psychology of personal experience, concerned with its development, its unconscious organization, and its therapeutic
transformation. Hence our next book (Atwood and
Stolorow, 1984), in which we developed the concept of an
intersubjective field as the fundamental theoretical construct for our framework, had as its subtitle *Explorations in
Psychoanalytic Phenomenology*.

If it was the investigation of the subjective origins of psychoanalytic theories that led us to phenomenology, it was the commitment to phenomenology, in turn, that led us ultimately to the recognition of a thoroughly contextualized subjectivity. Subjectivity, we came to realize, can only be the experience of a historically situated subject. To be an experiencing subject is to be positioned in the intersubjective contexts of past, present, and future. Husserl's phenomenological reduction is transformed into a phenomenological elaboration of complexity and process as properties of larger relational systems. Unremitting focus on the organization of personal experience, eschewing all isolated, reified mental entities, unveils the inescapable embeddedness of personal experience in constitutive intersubjective fields. Freud's ([1923] 1961a) intrapsychic determinism gives way to a thoroughgoing intersubjective contextualism.

In our view, the progression from phenomenology to contextualism was also a central feature in the development of Kohut's thought. Whereas we came to a phenomenological conception of psychoanalysis by examining the subjective origins of psychoanalytic theories, Kohut ([1959] 1978), unbeknownst to us, had earlier arrived at a similar conception by examining the relationship between mode of observation and theory in psychoanalysis. Beginning with the assumption that a scientific theory should be consistent with a science's method of investigation, Kohut reasoned that since the psychoanalytic method always includes introspection and empathy as its central constituents, only that which is in principle accessible to introspection and empathy belongs within the domain of psychoanalytic theory. Although he did not use these words, Kohut was essentially arguing here, much as we did later, that psychoanalytic theory should be a depth psychology of personal experience, because it is only personal experience and its vicissitudes that are accessible to the psychoanalytic method of investigation. Instinctual drive, for example, was to be expunged from psychoanalytic theory and replaced by the subjective experience of drivenness, which, we would add, is an affect state. However, with the exception of his (1977) reformulation of the oedipal phase, Kohut did not further pursue this focus on affect. In all three of his books (1971, 1977, 1984), he reverted to the concept of drives, although he relegated them increasingly to a subordinated role.

Still, Kohut's phenomenological emphasis did lead him to contextualism, although of a different form from ours. In order to understand the differences, let us return once again to the historical contexts.

At the time when our psychobiographical studies led us to phenomenology, we were academic psychologists interested in comparative personality theory. We were appalled by the fragmentation of the field of personality psychology into competing schools and doctrines, and we wanted to construct theoretical ideas of increasing generality and inclusiveness that could form the basis for a unifying framework. In our youthful expansiveness, we hoped that our psychoanalytic phenomenology—a framework that we believed was broad enough to encompass personal, subjective worlds in all their richness, diversity, and multidimensionality—would provide the foundation for a revolution in academic personality psychology whereby it could recover its lost commitment to studying human experience and conduct. Ironically, our ideas have had much greater influence in the field of clinical practice.

Kohut, in contrast, was not an academician, although he certainly could have been. He was a psychoanalytic clinician, who, in the mid-1960s, had come to focus specifically on the clinical problems of narcissism and narcissistic disorder. Therefore, the variant of contextualism to which Kohut was led by his turn to phenomenology was, in essence, a contextualization of narcissism, a theoretical contribution that opened a path, barred by Cartesian thought, to the psychoanalytic investigation and understanding of experiences of personal annihilation (see Chapter 8), and that significantly influenced our own clinical thinking. The concept of selfobject function (Kohut, 1971), in emphasizing that the organization of self-experience is always codetermined by the felt responsiveness of others, is a prime example of this contextualization. In Kohut's vision, narcissism and narcissistic disorder, no longer seen as products of the mechanics of an energy-disposal machine in which dammed-up libidinal cathexes are shunted to the haven of primordial solipsism, were revealed to be rooted in failures of caregivers to supply developmentally needed psychological nutriment, failures of human relationship. As a result of this contextualization of narcissism, the "windowless monads" of the philosopher Gottfried Leibniz were able to find some windows. The bad news, as we shall see, is that fundamentally they remained monads.

The clinical sensibility that followed from Kohut's contextualization of narcissism is well illustrated by his explicit attentiveness to the analyst's contribution to disruptions of the transference bond. Stormy transference reactions were grasped not as products of pathology located inside the patient's isolated mind but, in our language, as emergent properties of the patient-analyst system.

As useful and pathbreaking as his contextualization of narcissism may have been, Kohut's (1977) subsequent elevation of his psychology of narcissism to a metatheory of the total personality—a psychoanalytic psychology of the self—has created some knotty problems. For one thing, self psychology's unidimensionality, the exclusive focus on the narcissistic or selfobject dimension of experience and of transference—its establishment, disruption, and repair—has tended to become reductive, neglecting and failing to contextualize other important dimensions. Even more problematic has been the insidious movement from phenomenology to ontology, from experience to entities—a movement reminiscent of Freud's ([1923] 1961a) shift from the centrality of unconscious emotional conflict to the trinity of mental institutions presumed to explain it. In Kohut's jump from phenomenology to ontology, self as a fluidly evolving dimension of experience taking form within an ongoing contextual matrix is replaced by self as an objectified, supraordinate, agentic entity, an ontic being equipped with poles and a tension arc, and initiating actions to restore its own compromised cohesion. In this reification, which absolutized and universalized his clinical understandings, Kohut's hard-won contextualization of narcissism was partially undone, leading to an idolatry of psychological deficit, the doctrine of defects in the self (Orange, Atwood, and Stolorow, 1997). The Cartesian isolated mind returns here in the Romantic vision of a pristine nuclear self, with its inherent preprogrammed design, awaiting a responsive milieu that will enable it to unfold. Our view, by contrast, is that the trajectory of self-experience is shaped at every point in the life cycle by the intersubjective context in which it crystallizes. Phenomenology keeps us ever contextual.

As Howard Bacal and Kenneth Newman (1990) have pointed out, Kohut seemed reluctant to consider his framework a relational or two-person theory, probably because he wanted to preserve its link to the intrapsychic (and thus Cartesian) tradition of Freudian psychoanalysis and to prevent its being characterized as an interpersonal or social psychology. A post-Cartesian contextual psychology, by contrast, abolishes the persisting dichotomies between the intrapsychic and the interpersonal, between one-person and two-person psychologies, by recognizing that the individual and his or her world of personal experience are a subsystem of more encompassing relational or intersubjective suprasystems (Stolorow, 1997).

Next, we examine the epistemological dimension of psychoanalysis's movement toward contextualism. We have characterized this shift, in which the process itself of psychoanalytic knowing becomes contextualized, as a form of perspectivalism or perspectival realism (see Chapter 6). Cartesian isolated-mind thinking in psychoanalysis has historically been associated with a technical rationality (Orange, Atwood, and Stolorow, 1997) and an objectivist epistemology. That Kohut was a transitional figure in the movement of psychoanalytic thought from a Cartesian to a post-Cartesian epistemology is shown by the fact that some commentators—Robert Leider (1990) and Merton Gill (1994), for example—find evidence of objectivist attitudes in Kohut's writings, whereas others like ourselves

(Stolorow, 1990; Orange, 2000) have seen the leading edge of his thinking pointing toward perspectivalism. This latter trend is reflected in his assertion of an abiding belief in "the relativity of our perceptions of reality and . . . the relativity of the framework of ordering concepts that shape our observations and explanations" (Kohut, 1982, p. 400). In *How Does Analysis Cure?* (Kohut, 1984) he drew an explicit parallel between the shift from traditional analysis to self psychology and the shift from Newtonian physics to the Planckian physics of atomic and subatomic particles, in which "the field that is observed, of necessity, includes the observer" (p. 41), a point highly compatible with our own (Stolorow and Atwood, 1979) early emphasis on the indivisibility of the observer and the observed in the creation of psychoanalytic theories.

Despite these significant advances, remnants of a Cartesian objectivist epistemology persisted in Kohut's thinking, specifically in his conceptualizations of analytic empathy. Felicitously defining the proper analytic stance "as the responsiveness to be expected, on an average, from persons who have devoted their life to helping others with the aid of insights obtained via the empathic immersion into their inner life" (Kohut, 1977, p. 252), he unfortunately also claimed that such empathy "is in essence neutral and objective" (Kohut, 1980, p. 483), thereby decontextualizing it. The empathic stance could never be a neutral one because, like the traditional precepts of abstinence, anonymity, and equidistance, it is embedded in a theoretical belief system—one emphasizing the role of emotional responsiveness in facilitating the development of the sense of selfhood (Stolorow and Atwood, 1997). Furthermore, as Kohut (1980) himself well understood, "a situation in which one person has committed himself for prolonged periods to extend his 'empathic intention' toward another" (p. 487) is surely not experienced by the patient as a neutral one, meeting as it does deep longings to be understood.

It is the contention that the analyst's empathic immersions are objective that is especially saturated with Cartesian assumptions. One isolated mind, the analyst's, enters the subjective world of another isolated mind, the patient's, through the window, as it were. With his or her own psychological world virtually left outside, the analyst gazes directly upon the patient's inner experience with pure and preconceptionless eyes. From our vantage point, this doctrine of immaculate perception entails a denial of the inherently intersubjective nature of analytic understanding, to which the analyst's subjectivity makes an ongoing, unavertable contribution. To decenter (Piaget, [1970] 1974; Atwood and Stolorow, 1984) within a contextualist orientation means to become reflectively aware of how our analytic understandings are being influenced by our own personal organizing principles, not to banish these principles from the analytic system.

Donnel Stern (1997) has commented on the parallel between the differing epistemological stances of self psychology and relational psychoanalysis and the contrasting hermeneutical approaches of Friedrich Schleiermacher and Gadamer. Whereas Schleiermacher believed that a text can be interpreted by empathically entering the inner world of its author, Gadamer holds that such interpretation can only be from a perspective embedded in the historical matrix of the interpreter's own traditions.

Perspectivalism embraces the hermeneutical axiom that all human thought involves interpretation and that therefore our understanding of anything is always from a perspective shaped and limited by the historicity of our own organizing principles (Orange, Atwood, and Stolorow, 1997), by the fabric of preconceptions that Gadamer ([1975] 1991) calls "prejudice." The claim that all psychoanalytic understanding is interpretive means that there are no decontextualized absolutes or universals, no neutral or objective analysts, no immaculate perceptions, no God's-eye views (Putnam, 1990) of anything or anyone. This fallibilistic attitude (Chapter 6) encourages us to hold lightly not only theory but any particular view of meaning in the cocreated experience in the intersubjective field of treatment. It keeps our horizons open to multiple and expanding possibilities of meaning.

Our critical examination of Kohut's work is not intended as a devaluation of his contributions, which we regard as having deep historical significance and great clinical value. What we have criticized and sought to deconstruct is idolatry in its several guises. Idolatry forecloses dialogue, and, in a communitarian view of psychoanalytic knowing, it is dialogue above all else that will enable psychoanalytic theory to become ever more contextual, general, and inclusive.

5

Cartesian Trends
in Relational Psychoanalysis

*One of the greatest difficulties encountered in
bringing about favorable change is this almost
inescapable illusion that there is a perduring,
unique, simple existent self, [which is] in some
strange fashion, the patient's, or the subject
person's, private property.*

—**Harry Stack Sullivan**

During the past two decades, a number of viewpoints
have appeared that have sought, in varying degrees,
to emancipate psychoanalytic theory from Cartesian isolated-mind thinking. Among such evolving efforts to create a post-Cartesian psychoanalytic theory have been
Kohutian self psychology (Chapter 4), our own intersubjective systems theory (Stolorow and Atwood, 1992), and
American relational theory, as represented most prominently in the work of Stephen Mitchell and Aron.

Although Mitchell (1988) does not appear to have
been influenced by our earlier efforts to elaborate an intersubjective, contextualist perspective in psychoanalysis
(e.g., Atwood and Stolorow, 1984), his general descrip-

tion of relational-model theorizing is highly compatible with our viewpoint:

> In this vision the basic unit of study is not the individual as a separate entity . . . but an interactional field within which the individual arises and struggles to make contact and to articulate himself. *Desire* is experienced always *in the context of relatedness*, and it is that context which defines its meaning. Mind is composed of relational configurations. . . . Experience is understood as structured through interactions. (pp. 3–4, emphasis in original)

In a similar vein, Aron (1996) wrote:

> Relational theory is based on the shift from the classical idea that it is the patient's mind that is being studied (where mind is thought to exist independently and autonomously within the boundaries of the individual) to the relational notion that mind is inherently dyadic, social, interactional, and interpersonal. From a relational perspective, in investigating the mind the analytic process necessarily entails a study of the intersubjective field. (p. x)

In this chapter, we attempt to demonstrate that despite the important efforts of Mitchell, Aron, and other relational thinkers to recast psychoanalytic theory as a contextual psychology, relational psychoanalysis has, in significant ways, remained caught in the grip of the very Cartesianism it has sought to subvert. First we consider briefly the work of Sullivan and W. Ronald Fairbairn, theorists whose contributions are often cited as forerunners of contemporary relational theory. Then we question the "present-moment" thinking evident in much relational discourse. After discussing several influential conceptions of intersubjectivity, we next offer a critique of the concept of projective identification, a notion currently in vogue in relational circles. Lastly, we examine the mixed models prevalent in relational theorizing.

We wish to emphasize that among the works we critically review here are theoretical advances that have deep historical significance and great clinical value. Our critique is intentionally and avowedly one-sided, aimed not at a fair and balanced portrayal of the contributions under study but seeking instead to expose and challenge Cartesian assumptions hidden within even the most progressive of viewpoints. Indeed, we continue to search for such hidden assumptions in our own thinking. We are also aware that earlier important challenges to the Cartesianism of traditional psychoanalysis were made by "existential psychoanalysis" (see, for example, May, Angel, and Ellenberger, 1958). The existential analytic writers, however, tended to import into psychoanalytic theory concepts derived from isolated philosophical reflection—Heidegger's ([1927] 1962) ontological categories, for example—rather than grounding their ideas in the intersubjective dialogue of the psychoanalytic situation.

Sullivan

Interpersonal psychoanalysis grew out of Sullivan's (1950, 1953) attempt to replace the intrapsychic determinism of Freudian theory with an emphasis on the centrality of social interaction. Indeed, Sullivan wished to resituate psychiatry and psychoanalysis within the domain of the social sciences. His investigatory stance, however, vacillated between one that assumed a position *within* the experiential worlds of those involved in an interaction (an intersubjective perspective) and one that stood *outside* the transaction and presumed to make objective observations that were subject to "consensual validation." The latter stance is illustrated by Sullivan's concept of "parataxic distortion," a process through which a person's current experiences of others are said to be "warped" in consequence of his or her past interpersonal history. We wish to emphasize here that the concept of parataxic distortion enshrines a variant of the Cartesian doctrine of the isolated mind, a mind separated from an "objective" reality that it either accurately apprehends or distorts. This objectivist stance contrasts with a perspectival one, in which it is assumed that one's reality is *always* codetermined by features of the surround and the personal perspective from which these are viewed.

Fairbairn

The foundation stone of Fairbairn's (1952) metapsychology is his postulation of the motivational primacy of personal relatedness rather than instinctual discharge. Hence, libido for Fairbairn is always object seeking rather than pleasure seeking, relational rather than hedonic. Child-caregiver relationships undergo internalization, according to Fairbairn, only when they fail. The child adapts to depriving, ruptured, or traumatizing relationships by taking into himself or herself the badness of the needed other, thereby safeguarding the tie, preserving the hope of extracting love, and achieving the illusion of omnipotent control over the surround. An endopsychic world riddled with splits and repressions thus becomes established as a defensive and compensatory substitute for the faulty relationships with caregivers. Most important for the turn away from Cartesianism, from Fairbairn's viewpoint the basic structuralization of the psyche is seen as resulting from early patterns of experienced interaction with others. Psychological development is a property of the child-caregiver system.

Although Fairbairn highlighted the crucial importance of the surround in early developmental experiences—what Mitchell (1988) aptly termed the "developmental tilt"—in Fairbairn's theoretical vision, the endopsychic world, once established, is pictured as operating as a closed system, a Cartesian container housing an array of internalized personages. The internalized object relations are seen as dynamically active structures that behave at times like drives, at times like demons—autonomously and with a life of their own. Thus, in his view of the fully structuralized psyche, Fairbairn reverted to an image of the isolated mind, a mind whose dynamisms are insulated from the constitutive impact of the surround. In the analytic situation, this residual Cartesianism precluded the recognition and exploration of the part played by the analyst's personality, theoretical assumptions, and interpretive style in codetermining the evolution of the patient's transference experience.

Fairbairn's developmental theory strongly influenced the work of later object relations theorists. Otto Kernberg (1976), for example, has offered a revision of Freudian drive theory in which he pictures the basic building blocks of personality structure as units consisting of a self-image, an object image, and an affect. Units with a positive affective valence are said to coalesce into the libidinal drive, while those with a negative valence form the basis for the aggressive drive. Although Kernberg has acknowledged the early developmental and motivational importance of affect—another example of developmental tilt—once integrated into enduring self-object-affect units, affect states are seen to behave like drives, stirring within the confines of a Cartesian isolated mind and triggering all manner of distorting defensive activity. The lifelong embeddedness of affective experience in ongoing intersubjective systems thereby becomes lost.

Present-Moment Thinking

Among the various contexts considered in current relational discourse, by far the most prominent is the analysand-analyst dyad. Relational theorists like Mitchell (1988), Aron (1996), Irwin Hoffman (1983), and Owen Renik (1993) are not only providing extensive criticism of an exclusive theoretical and clinical focus on intrapsychic phenomena but are also advocating consistent attention to the analyst's contribution to clinical phenomena and to the formation and transformation of meanings. In our own work, we have insisted that analyst and patient form an indissoluble psychological system and that the organizing activities of both participants are crucial to understanding the meanings and impasses that develop in the intersubjective field. Thus, one crucial contextual consideration—the here and now—includes the interacting subjective worlds and organizing activities of both patient and analyst, including the analyst's theories and the cultural traditions of both participants.

Even a focus on dyadic context, however, can be vulnerable to residual Cartesianism in the form of atomism and atemporality. There is a tendency of some relational theorists (Gill, 1982; Mitchell, 1988) to privilege the here and now or snapshot context. They tend to deemphasize developmental contexts, as if serious consideration of these might infantilize the patient or create developmental tilt. Probably, their concern is a theoretical one that we share: Developmental thinking can easily become reductionistic or degenerate into mechanistic objectivism. If it does, we lose the complexity of psychological meanings, both found and formed in intersubjective systems, to a simplistic notion of causal genesis or etiology. We believe, however, that historical-developmental and cross-sectional contexts or dimensions cannot be neatly separated and that we must accord serious attention to their interpenetration. Ontologically, we regard the past and the future as inevitably implicated in all present moments (Bergson, [1910] 1960; Heidegger, [1927] 1962). Epistemologically, we find it impossible to know an isolated moment. Clinically, we find ourselves, our patients, and our psychoanalytic work always embedded in constitutive *process*. Process means temporality and history. To work contextually is to work developmentally. To work developmentally is to maintain a continuing sensibility to past, present, and future experience. Developmental thinking refuses the snapshot view—what Jacques Derrida (1978) and Jonathan Culler (1982) have called the "metaphysics of presence," or restriction to decontextualized moments or interactions—and affirms the emotional life of people who have come from somewhere and are going somewhere.

Unfortunately, serious attempts at relational theorizing can still slip into atomistic thinking. For example, Karen Maroda's (1991) courageous and thoughtful book on countertransference makes the following claim: "The only tenable position for us to adopt is to focus on the nature of interaction and the emotional states of the therapist and the patient *at the moment* to determine what approach is most helpful within the realm of what is genuine and humanly possible (p. 21)" (emphasis in original).

Without a developmental sensibility, a salutary emphasis on the personal presence and involvement of the analyst with the patient can lead to isolating the present moment. This present-moment thinking then becomes the new rule of technique, resulting in an overemphasis on what Renik (1999) has called an "ethic of self-disclosure" by analysts, or on the provision by analysts of what Morton Shane, Estelle Shane, and Mary Gales (1997) have described as "positive new experiences" not shaped by developmentally preformed organizing principles, as if experiences with no historicity, freeze-framed into an isolated moment, could ever be possible. The irony is that extremely well-intentioned and thoughtful attempts to understand clinical process in relational ways are undermined by antihistorical, decontextualized—and thus Cartesian—conceptions of human nature. Thinking contextually means ongoing sensitivity and relentless attention to a multiplicity of contexts—developmental, relational, gender-related, cultural, and so on (Orange, Atwood, and Stolorow, 1997).

Intersubjectivity and Mutual Recognition

The concept of intersubjectivity has become an important theme in current relational theorizing. Unfortunately, however, recent psychoanalytic discourse on intersubjectivity has been clouded by the intermixing and confounding of different uses of the term *intersubjective* that have distinctly different meanings at different levels of abstraction and generality. Developmentalists like Daniel Stern (1985) use the term *intersubjective relatedness* to refer to the developmental capacity to recognize another person as a separate subject. In a similar vein, Jessica Benjamin (1995), drawing on Hegel's ([1807] 1977) idea that self-consciousness is achieved through the reflection of one's consciousness in the consciousness of another, defines intersubjectivity as mutual recognition. Thomas Ogden (1994), by contrast, seems to equate intersubjectivity with what for us is only one of its dimensions, a domain of shared experience that is prereflective and largely bodily, what we call *unconscious nonverbal affective communication*. For us, intersubjectivity has a meaning that is much more general and inclusive, referring to the relational contexts in which all experience, at whatever developmental level, linguistic or prelinguistic, shared or solitary, takes form (Stolorow and Atwood, 1992). For us, an intersubjective field—any system constituted by interacting experiential worlds—is neither a mode of experiencing nor a sharing of experience. It is the contextual precondition for having any experience at all (Orange, Atwood, and Stolorow, 1997).

The Hegelian mutual-recognition model of intersubjectivity has led to a clinical emphasis on bringing the patient to a recognition of the subjectivity of the analyst, as if this goal defined the psychoanalytic process and could serve as a criterion of its success. Benjamin (1995), for example, has contended that "a theory in which the individual subject no longer reigns absolute must confront the difficulty each subject has in recognizing the other as an equivalent center of experience" (p. 28). Her mutual-recognition theory "postulates that the other must be recognized as another subject in order for the self to fully experience his or her subjectivity in the other's presence" (p. 30). To our ears, Benjamin's subjects, whether "the self" or "the other," sound very much like monadic Cartesian mind entities, with the exception that their objectification and separateness are not pregiven but achieved through an interactional process of mutual recognition.

In Benjamin's framework, fantasy is the antithesis of mutual recognition in that "all fantasy is the negation of the real other" (p. 45). This real other is defined as one "truly perceived as outside, distinct from our mental field of operations" (p. 29). Here we see a rather dramatic return of the Cartesian subject-object split, the separation of an absolutized external reality from a mind that perceives, distorts, or negates it. But according to whose decontextualized, preconceptionless God's-eye view (Putnam, 1990) do we say what is real and what is negation? Not even Jürgen Habermas ([1971] 1987), whose use of the term *intersubjectivity* Benjamin invoked, but whom she (1998) has faulted for not paying "sufficient attention to the subject's destructive omnipotence" (p. 93), would claim to know this definitively or in advance of a communicative process.

It would seem that residues of Melanie Klein's (1950b) idea of inherent destructiveness, perhaps made more palatable by Donald Winnicott ([1969] 1971), have evolved in some relational quarters into the notion of negation of the "real" other. Ogden (1994), another Hegelian Kleinian, defines psychoanalysis as "an effort to experience, understand, and describe the shifting nature of the dialectic generated by the creation and negation of the analyst by the analysand and of the analysand by the analyst" (p. 6). Benjamin's and Ogden's conceptualizations have in common a vision of substantialized Cartesian minds recognizing, creating, or negating one another. It would appear that Hegel's reflection model, so soundly criticized by twentieth-century phenomenologists and existentialists, has become for some relational psychoanalysts a way to exhort the aggressive Kleinian infant to become an ethical, less self-absorbed adult. One deleterious clinical consequence of such a hidden moral agenda is that psychoanalysis as questioning dialogue or making sense together (Orange, 1995) can degenerate into the analyst's imposing a demand for recognition upon the patient, with the latter's ability to do so being taken as a measure of analytic progress. Our own intersubjective systems theory, by contrast, imposes no such predetermined developmental outcome, except perhaps expansion of the patient's experiential horizons and enrichment of his or her affective life. In dynamic intersubjective systems, the outcomes of developmental or therapeutic processes are emergent and unforecastable rather than preprogrammed or prescribable (Stolorow, 1997).

Benjamin (1998) has recently declared that our viewpoint should be categorized as an interpersonal theory, thereby staking her claim to the term *intersubjective* for her own mutual-recognition theory. Yet interpersonal theorizing throughout its history has all too often been preoccupied with overt social behavior, the question of who is doing what to whom, such as the patient's provocations, manipulations, coercions, gambits, and the like. Our intersubjective perspective, by contrast, is not a theory of

behavioral interaction. It is a phenomenological field theory or dynamic systems theory that seeks to illuminate
interweaving worlds of experience. This was our meaning
of the term *intersubjective* when we first began using it
more than two decades ago (Stolorow, Atwood, and Ross,
1978).

Projective Identification

We view the notion of projective identification as one of
the last, seemingly unassailable strongholds of Cartesianism in relational psychoanalysis. Contemporary relational
theorists typically employ an interpersonalized version of
projective identification, in which Klein's (1950b)
description of a primitive fantasy is transformed into an
actual, causally efficacious interpersonal process through
which a person is presumed to translocate parts of himself
or herself into the psyche or soma of another. Consider, in
this regard, Kernberg's (1975) discussion of Ingmar
Bergman's movie *Persona:*

> A recent motion picture . . . illustrates the break-
> down of an immature but basically decent young
> woman, a nurse, charged with the care of a psy-
> chologically severely ill woman. . . . In the face of
> the cold, unscrupulous exploitation to which the
> young nurse is subjected, she gradually breaks
> down. . . . The sick woman seems to be able to live
> only if and when she can destroy what is valuable
> in other persons. . . . In a dramatic development,
> the nurse develops an intense hatred for the sick
> woman and mistreats her cruelly. . . . *It is as if all*
> *the hatred within the sick woman had been trans-*

ferred into the helping one, destroying the helping person from the inside. (pp. 245–246, emphasis added)

Here we see a caricature of the Cartesian isolated mind unleashed. A unidirectional influence system is pictured, wherein the subject's own omnipotent intrapsychic activity is claimed to create not only her own emotional experiences but the affective states of the other as well.

We have come to regard the doctrine of projective identification—the objectified image of one mind entity transporting its contents into another mind entity—as faithfully diagnostic of Cartesian isolated-mind thinking. Nevertheless, the concept, in one form or another, is an extremely popular one in current relational discourse. Mitchell (1988), for example, seems to have employed a variant of projective identification when he claimed that the analyst inevitably becomes a "coactor" in the patient's drama, "enacting the *patient's* old scenarios" (p. 293, emphasis in original) and inexorably falling into "the patient's predesigned categories" (p. 295). Ogden (1994) found that the concept of projective identification "provides essential elements" (p. 48) for his conception of intersubjectivity. Steven Stern (1994) chose projective identification as the theoretical linchpin for his "integrated relational perspective" (p. 317) on transference-countertransference enactments. Aron (1996) aptly criticized the notion of projective identification for portraying the analyst as an empty (Cartesian) container with no participating subjectivity of his or her own, but then referred approvingly to the concept's clinical utility.

Susan Sands (1997) has even proposed a marriage between the interpersonalized version of projective identification and Kohutian self psychology. As expounded by Sands, the theory of projective identification is invoked to "explain" those disquieting intersubjective situations in which the analyst feels "taken over" or "subjugated" by the patient's mind, as though there were an emotional "exchange of bodily fluids" whereby "the patient gets under the analyst's skin" (p. 663). It seems to us that what Sands is describing here are the analyst's visceral experiences of invasion, psychological usurpation, and self-loss, along with the fantasy the analyst uses to organize them. This fantasy attributes the analyst's disturbing experiences to the patient's unconscious intent. The theory of projective identification then objectifies and reifies the analyst's fantasy, transforming it into a real interpersonal process (or better, transpersonal process), whereby parts of the patient are presumed to be translocated into the analyst, much in the manner of a demonological possession. The tautological circle is now complete, as the patient is said to have "[taken] up residence inside the analyst" (p. 656) and to be "speaking to [the analyst] through [her] countertransference" (p. 654). The analyst feels invaded because she has, in fact, been taken over! In this respect, the theory of projective identification bears a striking resemblance to the delusion of the influencing machine (Tausk, 1917), which we (Orange, Atwood, and Stolorow, 1997) have understood as a vivid concretization of the experience of loss of personal agency resulting from extreme pathological accommodation (Brandchaft, [1993] 1994) to an alien will.

Roy Schafer (1972) long ago demonstrated how psychoanalytic formulations of mental actions like internalization and externalization employed reified fantasies of bodily incorporation and expulsion as pseudoexplanations of psychological processes, and we (Atwood and Stolorow, 1980) showed how such formulations involved an intermixing and a confusion of phenomenological (subjective) space with physical (objective) space. The theory of projective identification is a dramatic example of such confounding.

In addition to the errors of objectification and tautological circularity, there are other problems with the use of the concept of projective identification to explain the analyst's visceral states. There is, for example, the mistake of inferring causation from correlation. Because the analyst feels something that is also in the patient's experience in a not-yet-articulated form (correlation), it does not follow that the latter has produced the former (causation). It is equally plausible that there is a conjunction—an intersubjective correspondence—between regions of the patient's less articulated and the analyst's more articulated worlds of experience, a conjunction that creates the possibility of affective attunement. In general, the theory of projective identification wraps a cordon sanitaire around the analyst, obscuring the contribution of the analyst's organizing activity to the course of the therapeutic interaction.

Additionally, the model of causality reflected in the theory of projective identification is a linear one: X (the patient's hidden intent) causes Y (the analyst's visceral state). Increasingly, we are recognizing that grasping the vicissitudes of relational systems requires a nonlinear model of causality as offered by dynamic systems theory

(Stolorow, 1997). Patterns take form within a dynamic system through the intercoordination or cooperative interaction of its elements, following a trajectory unforecastable from any one element (e.g., the patient's unconscious intention) seen in isolation. We are not objecting here to the idea that patients may bring a hidden intentionality to the analytic encounter—only to the notion that such intentionality is the cause of, and can be directly inferred from, the analyst's visceral states.

There is more. The visceral states implicated in attributions of projective identification are states in which the experience and expression of affect have remained largely somatic—in which, that is, the affect has failed to evolve from its presymbolic, bodily form into symbolically articulated feelings. Yet the theory of projective identification presupposes the operation of highly developed symbolic processes—symbolizations of self, of other, and of the intended affective communications between them. The hidden intent to communicate—at the heart of the interpersonalized version of projective identification—presupposes the operation of symbolic thought. How can one intend to communicate experiences that have not yet been symbolized? Such a formulation is as untenable theoretically as Klein's (1950b) attribution of complex fantasy activity to presymbolic infants.

Tellingly, Sands (1997) has described the process of projective identification as occurring "in some mysterious way that we cannot begin to comprehend scientifically" (p. 653). We suggest, to the contrary, that the understanding of affective communication would be greatly enhanced by abandoning neo-Kleinian mysticism and demonology and turning instead to the laboratories of contemporary infant researchers. Beatrice Beebe, Frank Lachmann, and Joseph Jaffe (1997), for example, summarize the results of a highly relevant study by Nathan Fox (reported in Davidson and Fox, 1982), in which electroencephalograph (EEG) recordings were taken from ten-month-old infants viewing videotapes of faces displaying different affect states:

> If the infant is shown a videotape of a smiling-laughing actress, the pattern of EEG activation is one of positive affect; if the infant is shown a distressed, crying actress, the pattern of EEG activation is one of negative affect. The infant cannot escape the emotion of the partner as reflected on the partner's face. (Beebe, Lachmann, and Jaffe, 1997, p. 143)

Surely no one would argue that the affects from the videotapes got under the infants' skin and into their brains because of the taped faces' unconscious intent to communicate these states to the babies. The Fox study demonstrates that infants are prewired to participate in nonverbal affective communication. Any assumptions about unconscious intentionality or projective mechanisms presumed to explain such communication are entirely unwarranted.

Because we are contextualists, it is our belief that the meanings embedded in a theoretical idea cannot be fully comprehended without examining its historical and personal contexts of origin. Klein's (1950b) metapsychology, of which projective identification is an integral component, is a monadic drive theory that accounts for psychological life in terms of the workings of an innate aggressive drive located deep within an isolated mind. The theory of projective identification can be viewed as an attempt to escape this self-encapsulated isolation and to find some form of communicative connection with a fantasized other. The result is a portrait of two decontextualized Leibnizian windowless monads trying to create windows. Kleinian theory, no matter how much it is interpersonalized, is drenched in Cartesian presuppositions.

Why is it that the concept of projective identification has been so successful in getting under the skin of psychoanalysis? One reason is that the concept allows therapists and analysts to disavow unwanted aspects of their own affectivity, attributing them to unconscious projective mechanisms originating in the mind of the patient. In effect, the theory of projective identification does to the patient exactly what the theory says the patient is doing to the clinician. The demon of projective identification, a stubbornly persisting relic of Cartesianism, needs to be cast out if relational theory is to become more fully contextual.

Mixed Models

Mixed models that perpetuate, rather than subvert, the original Cartesian division between outer and inner realms are prevalent in contemporary relational theorizing. Emmanuel Ghent (1992), for example, stated that from a relational viewpoint, "both reality and fantasy, both outer world and inner world, both the interpersonal and the intrapsychic, play immensely important and interactive roles in human life" (p. xviii). Similarly, Aron (1996) saw "relational theory as maintaining both one- and two-person psychologies" (p. 47), existing in a complementary and dialectical relationship. This dialectical perspective, according to Aron, allows relational psychoanalysis to achieve a "balance between internal and external relationships, real and imagined relationships, the intrapsychic and the interpersonal, the intrasubjective and the intersubjective, the individual and the social" (p. ix). Accordingly, although claiming that abandonment of drive theory is central to relational psychoanalysis, he allowed drives and the isolated mind to slip in through the back door in the form of "inherent motivations" (p. 47), such as universal strivings for union and separateness, or in the guise of preprogrammed developmental stages imported from Freudian and Kleinian theory.

Aron has even attempted to resuscitate the Cartesian dinosaur of objectivity by proposing for psychoanalysis an objectivity that is "dialectical and dialogical" (p. 263), a glaring oxymoron from our point of view and from the standpoint of his own perspectivalism. More recently, Marvin Wasserman (1999) has proposed an "integrated stance" that combines elements from both one-person and two-person psychologies, whereby the analyst "retains neutrality, anonymity, and abstinence as analytic ideals, recognizing that they can never be fully achieved" (p. 454).

It is our view that the persisting dichotomies between the intrapsychic and the interpersonal, between one-person and two-person psychologies, are obsolete—reified, absolutized relics of the Cartesian bifurcation. The very phrase *two-person psychology* continues to embody an atomistic, isolated-mind philosophy in that two separated mental entities, two thinking things, are seen to bump into each other. We ought to speak instead of a contextual psychology, in which experiential worlds and intersubjective fields are seen as equiprimordial, mutually constituting one another in circular fashion. Unlike Cartesian isolated minds, experiential worlds, as they form and evolve within a nexus of living, relational systems, are recognized as being exquisitely context-sensitive and context-dependent. In this conception, the Cartesian subject-object split is mended, and inner and outer are seen to interweave seamlessly. We inhabit our experiential worlds even as they inhabit us. Mind is pictured here as an emergent property of the person-environment system, not as a Cartesian entity localized inside the cranium.

Ghent, Aron, and Wasserman, like many other relationally oriented psychoanalysts, are caught between two incompatible philosophical worlds. One is the world Freud inherited from Descartes, a world of Archimedean certainty and clear objectivity, in which isolated-mind entities are radically estranged from external others. The other is the world of post-Cartesian contextualism, which recognizes the constitutive role of relatedness in the making of all experience. Relational theorists have tried to combine, reconcile, and preserve elements of these two worlds by claiming that they can coexist in some form of dialectical relationship. We believe that such efforts, although appealing, cannot succeed, because these two philosophical worlds are fundamentally incommensurable. We must choose.

Yet, as we have seen, remnants of Cartesian isolated-mind thinking persist, even in the works of authors who have argued eloquently and persuasively for their deconstruction. As suggested in Chapter 1, the reasons for such persistence are more psychological than philosophical. Aron (1996) alluded to a partial explanation in his reference to Bernstein's (1983) concept of "Cartesian anxiety," what we have termed "the fear of structureless chaos" (Stolorow, Atwood, and Brandchaft, 1994, p. 203). Without reified mental entities, without decontextualized absolutes or universals, and without objectivity and its God's-eye view, we are left with no metapsychological or epistemological bedrock to stand on, and the resulting anxiety can be enormous. In order not to retreat into the reassuring illusions of Cartesianism, we must find ways to embrace the painful vulnerability inherent in "the unbearable embeddedness of being" (Stolorow and Atwood, 1992, p. 22), especially as this vulnerability is evoked in our psychoanalytic work. Even experiences of discreteness and individuality, absolutized by the Cartesian bifurcation, are embedded in constitutive context.

We wish to emphasize, however, that contextualism in psychoanalysis should not be confused with postmodernist nihilism or relativism, as some critics (e.g., Bader, 1998; Leary, 1994) have done. Relativity to context is not the same thing as a relativ*ism* (Orange, 1995) that considers every framework, whether psychoanalytic or moral, to be as good as the next. Pragmatically, some ideas are better than others in facilitating psychoanalytic inquiry and the psychoanalytic process. Moreover, we do not abandon the search for truth, for lived experience, for subjective reality. We hold that closer and closer approximations of such truth are gradually achieved through a psychoanalytic dialogue in which the domain of reflective self-awareness is enlarged for both participants. And here we arrive at a fundamental tenet of our post-Cartesian contextualism: Truth is dialogic, crystallizing from the inescapable interplay of observer and observed.

Part Two

Clinical Implications

6

Perspectival Realism
and Intersubjective Systems

It makes a difference whose ox is gored.
—**Martin Luther**

*The person with understanding does not know
and judge as one who stands apart and unaf-
fected; but rather, as one united by a specific
bond with the other, he thinks with the other
and undergoes the situation with him.*
—**Hans-Georg Gadamer**

In this chapter, we examine the relationship between our
intersubjective systems theory and an epistemological
attitude that one of us (Orange, 1995) has termed *perspectival realism*. Our argument exemplifies the more general proposition that a focus on complexity and the
dynamics of complex systems coincides with a perspectival
view of knowing (Cilliers, 1998). The link we are sug-
gesting between psychoanalytic intersubjectivity theory
and our version of perspectivalism holds important clinical
implications that we also discuss here.

As we noted in Chapter 4, the early germs of our
intersubjective contextualism can be found in a series of

psychobiographical studies, collected in our first book (Stolorow and Atwood, 1979), exploring the personal, subjective origins of four psychoanalytic theories. Although neither the concept of intersubjectivity nor a perspectivalist epistemology was explicitly introduced in the first edition of this book, both were implicit in the demonstrations of how the subjective world of a psychological theorist profoundly influences his or her understanding of others' experiences. These studies led us to a phenomenological conception of psychoanalysis and, in turn, to the recognition of a thoroughly contextualized subjectivity—of the inescapable embeddedness of personal experience in constitutive context.

The phrase *intersubjective perspective* first appeared in a work written by our group some twenty-five years ago (Stolorow, Atwood, and Ross, 1978), an article that Aron (1996) credited with having introduced the concept of intersubjectivity into American psychoanalytic discourse. This article explored the impact on the therapeutic process of correspondences and disparities (conjunctions and disjunctions) between the subjective worlds of patient and analyst. In the years that followed, our intersubjective perspective evolved into a field theory or dynamic systems theory that comprehends psychological phenomena not as products of isolated intrapsychic mechanisms but as forming at the interface of reciprocally interacting worlds of experience. It is not the isolated individual mind, we have repeatedly argued, but the larger system created by the mutual interplay between the subjective worlds of patient and analyst, or of child and caregiver, that constitutes the domain of psychoanalytic inquiry.

The psychoanalytic doctrine of intrapsychic determinism, a direct descendant of Descartes's worldless subject and subjectless world, has historically been associated with an objectivist epistemology. Such a position envisions the mind in isolation, radically estranged from an external reality that it either accurately apprehends or distorts. Analysts embracing an objectivist epistemology presume to have privileged access both to the patient's psychic reality and to the objective truths it distorts. In contrast, our intersubjective viewpoint, emphasizing the constitutive interplay between worlds of experience, is inextricably melded to a perspectivalist epistemology. This epistemological attitude presumes neither that the analyst's subjective reality is more true than the patient's nor that the analyst can directly know the subjective reality of the patient; the analyst can only approximate the patient's subjective reality from within the particularized and delimited horizons of the analyst's own perspective. A perspectivalist attitude has a profound effect on the ambience of the psychoanalytic situation, the subject to which we now turn.

Clinical and Philosophical Reflections

"I have been so upset," a longtime patient begins. "I can't get out of my head that you called me a borderline. I can't stop thinking that that is what I really am and that that is how you see me." "Oh, no," the analyst thinks, "it's not possible. I have a poor memory, but I couldn't have. I don't even believe in the borderline concept and cannot remember ever having called anyone by that name." So the analyst says to her patient that what she has done to him is terrible and asks him to tell her when it happened and what they had been talking about. She acknowledges that his memory is generally much better than hers.

Another patient says that she assumes the analyst's political views differ from hers (she was raised Marxist) and that the analyst will therefore be unable to understand her or to take her seriously. "Granted," she continues, "you do seem mostly to understand me and to have compassion for my troubles, but it couldn't be real respect if we don't really agree." The analyst imagines herself, of course, to be reasonably capable of at least adequately understanding those with whom she disagrees and of having considerable respect for people who hold different opinions.

A third patient believes the analyst is relieved to be away from him when she is away on professional or personal travels and tells her this on his way out the door. She is unaware of the feeling he attributes to her, but his conviction about this is so strong that he cannot imagine any other possibility. So where are reality and truth in clinical work?[1]

---

[1] In most philosophical discourse, questions of reality concern ontological status, that is, the existence or nonexistence of mind, matter, concepts, worlds, and so on, that may exist independently of any knowledge or opinion about them. So, for example, Galileo—until imprisoned and threatened with worse—claimed that the earth *really* moved around the sun whether the Roman cardinals thought so or not. Truth and falsehood, by contrast, concern the status of beliefs or sentences and, in contemporary philosophy, whole systems of beliefs upon which the meaning and truth of a particular belief depends. Galileo clearly thought that his research and observations gave him access to more, or at least different, truth than that derived from revelation. Theories of truth—correspondence, coherence, pragmatic—concern the putative connections between truth and reality. A scientific worldview like that of Galileo and most psychoanalysts (Orange, 1995) usually relies on a pragmatic theory of truth that combines elements of the correspondence and coherence theories.

We introduce these rather ordinary clinical instances, not to illustrate not-always-brilliant clinical work or to prove the "truth" of a particular psychoanalytic theory but rather to serve as reference points for a reclarification of our perspectival realism (Orange, 1995), to show how well this epistemology suits an intersubjective systems view of psychoanalysis, and to suggest that epistemologies have clinical consequences.

In each of the three clinical stories, the patient and analyst have points of view that differ considerably. In the first, the analyst's impulse is simply to say that the patient is wrong, mistaken, or even delusional. She simply cannot have done what she is accused of. In the second, the analyst grants the premise (she has never been a Marxist and is therefore somewhere to the right of the patient politically). This "reality" they both recognize. The analyst does not, however, believe as the patient does that true understanding and respect between them are therefore impossible. She is tempted to say the patient is wrong, mistaken, biased, and unnecessarily hopeless. In the third instance, the particular patient who says his analyst will be relieved to get away from him is *not* one by whom she is aware of feeling burdened. So she is tempted to say he is wrong, mistaken, perhaps paranoid or projecting. In each case, the temptation is to say, or at least to feel, that the analyst is right and that the patient has poor reality testing.

We deliberately choose such commonplace examples and such ordinary temptations, which, we assume, thoughtful and experienced analysts of all theoretical persuasions try to resist. We have learned to hesitate and to ask ourselves whether matters could actually be so simple.

We have learned to recognize that many such statements by patients injure our sense of professional selfhood and that we may thus be too readily inclined to react by pathologizing the patient's perspective. We have learned to wonder about the meanings the assertion in question could have for the patient. Still, we analysts also seem to participate in a common human propensity to see one's own perspective as the measure of truth and rather automatically to judge those with whom we disagree as unrealistic and misguided. This tendency is sometimes supported by the claim that philosophical discussions about reality are irrelevant to our work.

A recent article by Lawrence Friedman (1999), for example, claimed to show that "the philosophical problem that is reached for is really an unfamiliar one, arcane, irresolvable, and not especially relevant to psychoanalysis" (p. 401). Friedman described the growth of modern objectivist epistemology as well as the skeptical reaction against it (there *really* is no truth or reality). Then, to our surprise, he claimed that this whole discussion has nothing to offer to psychoanalysis.

> It is sometimes said that the reason we feel uneasy talking about reality in our work is that we now realize that there is no state of affairs existing independent of the way we think about it. We are urged to bring psychoanalysis up to date by abandoning the illusion that there is an objective truth that can be pursued, discovered, and authoritatively pronounced upon. This error is often called "positivism." The cure is supposed to be the sophisticated philosophy of the twentieth century. . . . Properly

identified, the problem that really bedevils analytic theorists is not the notion of objective reality per se, but the notion of an objective *social* or *human* reality, which is the way the problem has traditionally been identified in psychoanalysis. If analysts could sort out that concept and say what social reality is, reality in general would pose no special challenge and we would not have to submit to radical skepticism. (pp. 401–402)

We should instead, he suggested, concern ourselves with something more mundane and truly psychoanalytic: what he calls *realisticness*, "the ability to sample human meaning from several affective and cognitive perspectives" (p. 418), versus "unrealisticness." The outcome of a good analysis, he declared, is an increase of realisticness. In Friedman's view, philosophical discussions have no bearing on this distinction; psychoanalysis and philosophy as disciplines are separate and should remain so. In his words, "Psychoanalysis need not concern itself with every philosophical problem. We should not accept philosophical bullying without assurance that the hoary question invoked is truly and especially germane to psychoanalysis" (p. 421).

Friedman's understanding that scientific empiricism/ logical positivism undermined commonsense realism and thus set the conceptual stage for the currently fashionable postmodern skepticism (pp. 404–406) is an insight rarely found even among philosophers. In Friedman's words, "With impressive intelligence and workmanship, the positivists had painstakingly honed a precise language in which the entire world would be derived from provable, individual experiences, only to end up with no world, no experience, and nothing but a free choice of arbitrary language systems" (p. 406). Friedman has written us a cogent history of the disputes about reality and truth but has then thrown it all away.

We think Friedman's position is undermined, first, by his identification of the current critique of objectivist thinking with the skeptical relativism of Nietzsche ([1886] 1973), Jean-François Lyotard (1984), and Richard Rorty (1989) and, second, by his characterization of philosophical questioning as "bullying." The more moderate post-Cartesian critiques developed by pragmatists like Hilary Putnam (1990) and Bernstein (1983), as well as Continental philosophies like the communicative praxis of Habermas ([1971] 1987) and the hermeneutics of Gadamer ([1975] 1991), offer rich possibilities for understanding and articulation in psychoanalysis. In fact, Friedman's own description of his "realisticness" could easily be contextualized and grounded with reference to these latter thinkers.

Otherwise we must ask, "realisticness" according to whom? From whose perspective? Yes, there is really an elephant in the old fable (see parable at the end of this chapter), but which perspective or combination of perspectives is realistic? No one can take all perspectives, the God's-eye view (Putnam, 1990). Perhaps all of us, and not only patients, have blind spots. Has the patient become realistic when she or he comes to agree with the analyst in the sampling of perspectives? Or with the majority (consensual validation)? What happens to minority opinion? Does it belong on the trash heap of delusion? And what is delusion? Do not our concepts of delusion and also of psychosis depend upon the assumption that there is a privileged point of view not limited by perspective? We believe that we psychoanalysts need philosophical reflection to help us with these questions. Victoria Hamilton (1993) has studied the implicit epistemological positions taken by psychoanalysts of various theoretical persuasions, and her results imply that there is commonly no explicitly acknowledged connection between a psychoanalyst's epistemological assumptions and his or her theory. Philosophy is not a subject-matter discipline like chemistry or sociology or history, clearly distinguishable from the contents and methods of psychoanalysis. Philosophy is the process of making both our unacknowledged presuppositions and the limitations of our perspectives explicit so that we can question each other and ourselves.

Perspectival Realism

For a post-Cartesian psychoanalytic praxis, one of us has proposed (Orange, 1995) that we approach the question of reality in psychoanalysis by way of a perspectival realism, seeing truth as gradually emergent in dialogic community:

> Each participant in the inquiry has a perspective that gives access to a part or an aspect of reality. An infinite—or at least an indefinite—number of such perspectives is possible. . . . Since none of us can entirely escape the confines of our personal perspective, our view of truth is necessarily partial, but conversation can increase our access to the whole. . . . Perspectival realism recognizes that the only truth or reality to which psychoanalysis provides access is the subjective organization of experience understood in an intersubjective context. . . . Such

a subjective organization of experience is one perspective on a larger reality. We never fully attain or
know this reality but we continually approach,
apprehend, articulate, and participate in it. . . .
While this view does exclude common-sense
realisms, correspondence theories of truth, and scientific empiricisms, it does not exclude the possibility of dialogic, communitarian, or perspectival
realism. In such a moderate realism, the real is an
emergent, self-correcting process only partly accessible via personal subjectivity but increasingly
understandable in communitarian dialogue. (pp.
61–62)

This is not an original idea. It has extensive roots in philosophy and is shared by many psychoanalysts who are
currently articulating various senses of its extensive clinical
relevance.

The question of philosophical roots needs to be
approached with some care. Nietzsche ([1886] 1973) is
the philosopher most associated with a radical perspec-
tivism. His railing against what he saw as the absolutes of
Enlightenment rationalism led him to advocate revaluing
all values, transcending good and evil, and glorifying irra-
tionality. For him, and even more for his "postmodern"
and "neopragmatist" admirers, there is nothing but perspective. Although this is the Nietzsche who has come
down to us through Heidegger and the French postmod-
ernists, we think there may be another, less appreciated,
gadfly Nietzsche, perhaps valued by Freud, who
attempted to shock us out of our philosophical and religious unconsciousness.

Our own influences, on the contrary, include early phenomenologists such as Franz Brentano ([1874] 1973) and Husserl ([1931] 1962, [1936] 1970), for whom a perspective always means a perspective on something (intentionality). There is no "view from nowhere" (Nagel, 1986), but neither is there perspective without something (an elephant, perhaps) on which to take a point of view. In addition, we are indebted for our pragmatic realism to American philosopher Peirce ([1905] 1931–1935), whose "concrete reasonableness" captures, we think, the idea Friedman has searched for in psychoanalysis. Peircean fallibilism expresses the attitude that there is always something more to be learned and that our own perspective is limited and therefore mistaken insofar as we take it to be the whole truth. The advocates of dialogic understanding and of communicative praxis—Gadamer ([1975] 1991) and Habermas ([1971] 1987), respectively—are further influences. Most recently, in Wittgenstein's (1953) therapeutic conception of philosophy, we have found further inspiration for our perspectival realism. Let us consider each in turn.

Our perspectival realism owes its insistence on intentionality to Brentano, teacher of both Husserl and Freud (the young Freud, who later disavowed interest in philosophy, was so impressed by Brentano that he took five courses from him). For Brentano, intentionality meant that mental activity is by nature directional, that is, that thinking means thinking *something*, that desiring means desiring *something*, and so on. As we understand it, intentionality implies that taking a perspective or point of view means taking a point of view on or toward *something*. Brentano's intentionality, stripped of his early claim that

the object is immanent in the thought, forms an important element in our view that emphasis on the plurality of
perspectives is compatible with what Putnam (1990)
called "realism with a human face." Although Brentano's
Aristotelian realism would have excluded him from postmodernism, he had no use for dogmatisms. A Catholic
priest, he left the church after 1871 because he could not
accept the doctrine of papal infallibility. Although perspectival realism is our phrase, not his, we could say that,
for him, papal infallibility implied that *one* perspective
contained absolute and total truth.

The American philosopher and logician Peirce was
likewise horrified by the claim of papal infallibility, so
much so that he proclaimed that his own thinking, and all
respectable science, must be fallibilist, capable of error,
and open to revision. He is best known, however, and
clearly acknowledged by William James ([1898] 1975), as
the originator of American pragmatism, carefully articulated by him in this way: "Consider what effects, that
might conceivably have practical bearings, we conceive the
object of our conception to have. Then, our conception of
these effects is the whole of our conception of the object"
(Peirce, [1905] 1931–1935, vol. 5, para. 402). Peirce's
pragmatism, changed beyond recognition by William
James's popularizations and then renamed by Peirce
"pragmaticism, which is ugly enough to be safe from kid-
nappers" (Peirce, [1905] 1931–1935, vol. 5, para. 414),
forms the kernel of our sense that ideas are equivalent to
their conceivable practical consequences. It is therefore
amazing to us to hear well-educated psychoanalysts say
that they have no interest in ideas, but only in clinical
cases. (We have had journal submissions and conference

papers rejected on precisely these grounds.) Like Peirce, and now Habermas, whose Peircean views are sometimes called "language-pragmatic intersubjectivity" (Frank, 1991), we believe that practice and ideas are inextricable from each other. Analysts' theoretical ideas are just as integral to their being as are the emotional convictions of both patient and analyst (Stolorow and Atwood, 1979). These concepts affect our clinical practice—one need only see patients treated by analysts of various theoretical orientations to realize this—and thus deserve our careful philosophical questioning. (Indeed, we would suggest that Friedman's own attempt to articulate a workable concept of "realisticness" is a form of philosophical reflection.) Altogether, Peirce's pragmatism, his fallibilism, and his ideal of truth-seeking within a community of scholars have significantly shaped our convictions about psychoanalysis as theory-formed practice—as clinical philosophy, as it were.

A further influence is Gadamer, whose hermeneutic concept of dialogic understanding significantly underlies our sense of the day-to-day and moment-to-moment process in psychoanalysis. For him, any truth arises from the interplay of perspectives, each carrying its load of tradition and preconceptions:

> In reading a text, in wishing to understand it, what we always expect is that it will *inform* us of something. A consciousness formed by the authentic hermeneutical attitude will be receptive to the origins and entirely foreign features of that which comes to it from outside its own horizons. Yet this receptivity is not acquired with an objectivist

"neutrality": it is not possible, not necessary, and not desirable that we put ourselves within brackets. The hermeneutical attitude supposes only that we self-consciously designate our opinions and prejudices and qualify them as such, and in so doing strip them of their extreme character. In keeping to this attitude we grant the text the opportunity to appear as an authentically different being and to manifest its own truth, over and against our own preconceived notions. (Gadamer, [1975] 1991, pp. 151–152)

Here we see several aspects of a hermeneutic attitude that contribute to perspectival realism as a psychoanalytic epistemology. To begin with, there is the assumption that there is something under discussion: for "the text," we may substitute the patient's history, the patient's suffering, a misunderstanding between patient and analyst, or the heating or cooling system in the analyst's office. This something makes its own demands on the discussion and requires us to identify and recognize our own preconceptions and thus "strip them of their extreme character." We are thus able to recognize our own view as a perspective, so that the matter itself *(die Sache selbst)* can show up as other. In addition, of course, we can hear our patients and colleagues as having access to realities that are hidden from us by our own perspective—this is what it means to be other. We should always expect, according to Gadamer, that the other text or person can teach us something. In his thinking, Peircean fallibilism becomes the receptivity to the perspectives of others. Our limited perspective leaves us likely to be at least partly wrong, because we are tempted to take our own opinion or view as a fair account of the whole. Only in playful dialogue with people or texts or works of art (this includes serious discussion of serious matters) do we have the opportunity to overcome this severe limitation of the solitary apprehension of anything and allow more truth, truth-as-possible-understanding (Frank, 1992), to emerge.

Habermas has added an ethical dimension to our thinking about the problems of reality and truth in psychoanalysis. For him, political justice depends on conversation between participants assumed to be interested in reasonable solutions to the problems of the community. The only just society is one that respects its different voices and perspectives and assumes that no one voice (here we must hear his "never again") possesses the truth or the accurate apprehension of reality. A similar note has been sounded in American psychoanalysis by Janice Gump (2000) in her challenge to the racial exclusion and blindness in American psychoanalysis. Voices and perspectives absent from the conversation significantly reduce our access to realities and truths.

Finally, reading Wittgenstein has confirmed our sense that the questions of truth and of meaning are importantly distinct. Meanings can only exist within a culture, a language game, or a form of life. A language game, for Wittgenstein, is a rule-guided activity, similar to chess, in which the meanings of words arise from their use within the game. There is no meaning-in-itself. All the words and all the moves in the game are meaningless apart from the system. There is an irreducible plurality of these language games, but our failure to distinguish them from one another, for instance, by mixing everyday and philosophical questions, leads to endless confusion. According to Wittgen-stein, the task of a philosopher is to point out these pitfalls.

If we are playing chess, we can identify the exact location of the king on the game board, without reference to the rules of the game. It is true to say that the king is really in such-and-such a place. If we are engaging in psychoanalysis, we can likewise distinguish between questions of meaning and those of truth. The meaning questions arise within the field created by the interplay of the analyst's and the patient's subjective worlds, including the analyst's theories. They also arise as a consequence of the inevitable difference in perspective between the two worlds.

Consider, for example, the fee, a feature of most psychoanalyses. Its meanings differ, depending on whose perspective we are considering, the meanings of money in a given culture, the similarity or difference of economic class between patient and analyst, and so on. Truth and reality are not at stake here: The fee is what it is, in the currency of a given country at a given time, just as the king in chess is located wherever it is. But this reality and our true belief in it give rise to many possibilities of meaning and of understanding reached between the people involved.

Wittgenstein never disputed the reality of commonly agreed upon states of affairs, for example, that England and Austria were in different parts of Europe. He did attempt to get us to see that such statements, true as they may be, only have meaning within the systems of communication he called language games. So we claim his support for our claim that there is reality, but that perspective and culture limit our knowing of it, that statements of truth or falsehood are meaningful only within systems, and that conversation is required for meanings to become apparent. The process of making sense together of whatever we find we call *understanding*.

Perspectival Realism in Clinical Work

We often say that there are three indispensable components to an intersubjective clinical sensibility. First is the focus on organizing principles, central themes, or emotional convictions that characterize a person's experiential world.

> The principal components of subjectivity, in our view, are the organizing principles, whether automatic and rigid, or reflective and flexible. These principles, often unconscious, are the emotional conclusions a person has drawn from lifelong experience of the emotional environment, especially the complex mutual connections with early caregivers. Until these principles become available for conscious reflection, and until new emotional experience leads a person to envision and expect new forms of emotional connection, these old inferences will thematize the sense of self. This sense of self includes convictions about the relational consequences of possible forms of being. A person may feel, for example, that any form of self-articulation or differentiation will invite ridicule or sarcasm. (Orange, Atwood, and Stolorow, 1997, p. 7)

Working with these emotional convictions as they emerge in various forms in our work is the bread and butter of intersubjective systems work in psychoanalysis.

Without our second component, self-reflexivity, we could easily be misunderstood as saying that these organizing principles are the contents of isolated minds, simply substituted for the Freudian drives and their derivatives. We must hasten to say, therefore, that an intersubjective clinical sensibility requires the empathic connection of which Gadamer so eloquently speaks as "undergoing the situation" with the other. Self-reflexivity, as we use the term, means two things. First is a constant awareness of our presence, with all our history and prejudices, in the process of understanding the other. There is no immaculate perception or pure empathic immersion. The best we can do is a relentless search for understanding of the emotional predicaments in which we are ourselves implicated and that we can only hear with our own particular ears. Second, aware that our theories embody our own historically shaped emotional convictions and themes, we must hold lightly whatever perspective we may have on the patient's troubles and remain ready to question our cherished psychoanalytic theories of human nature with their associated views of psychopathology and cure.

To come back to the theme of this chapter, the third component of an intersubjective sensibility is that there will be no arguments about reality. Reality is whatever it is, but as analysts our task is to hold our own perspectives as lightly as we can so that the other's words can speak to us. Returning to the example given at the beginning of this chapter, it is really not important whether the analyst used the word "borderline" or not. This word was her patient's way of pointing to the reality that something had gone very wrong between them, and the analyst's instant denial—verbally expressed or not—signaled her unawareness of what had happened. We must attend to truth-as-possible-understanding and not truth-as-correspondence-to-fact. Whatever the facts may be, we must find ways to converse about the meanings, and arguments about reality and the associated insistence that the patient recognize the analyst's perspective are usually the quickest exits from the search for understanding. In this instance, the analyst had sounded to this patient as if she were being reductive (classifying) and demeaning of his experience. She had to recognize that she had been carried away in a "I am so smart and I can tell you what the trouble is" moment. Since the patient had grown up in a home where the *DSM* (psychiatry's *Diagnostic and Statistical Manual*) was the family dictionary, the story came out in these words. But this was not important. What helped was for the analyst to acknowledge that she had set herself in a know-it-all position vis-à-vis her patient and that this had caused actual harm, if only temporary, to their connection and to their joint search for emotional understanding.

Likewise with the Marxist, the analyst had to ask herself what was true in the patient's point of view and try to put her own view in the background. If the analyst had defensively argued that differences are compatible with respect, she would have completely lost what this patient was trying to tell her. In this case, the patient's gradual loss of her Marxist world—the only one in which she had ever felt like a somebody—had meant an irreparable loss of her sense that she belonged in any world at all, and she was terrified that the analyst, like all the others, could not see her as valuable. They came to understand that the patient's growing attachment to her analyst had evoked a panicky conviction that this could only mean more loss and humiliation.

As for the third patient, the analyst immediately denied that she was relieved to be away from him. Of course, this was not very much help. All he could say was, "I know I'm crazy." This incident occurred, fortunately, more than one session before the analyst's travels, so she was able to respond, "This is important; let's be sure to talk about it next time," her usual reassurance to the patient that she has heard him and to herself that surely she can do better work. In fact, neither of them really wanted to talk about it next time, but they did. It turned out that something about the way their sessions had been ending (related to a change in the analyst's schedule) had given this patient, already feeling unwanted and a burden to anyone he cared for, the feeling that she was glad to see him go. Talking about this pattern between them and about the analyst's awareness of her own need to be a good caregiver (she is the oldest of ten siblings) showed her how blinded by her perspective she had been to his experience of their relationship. Her refraining from arguing about reality, combined with the self-reflexive awareness mentioned earlier, together with interest in the convictions organizing the experience of each of them and both of them together, allowed them to progress along the path of truth-as-possible-understanding.

In summary, although this chapter has as its primary concern the articulation of perspectival realism as a fruitful philosophical position and attitude for psychoanalysis, it has also been concerned with all three components of an intersubjective clinical sensibility. Indeed, we have tried to show that a perspectivalist epistemology and our intersubjective perspective go hand in hand. We have also attempted to distinguish here between the reality of what is undeniable within particular systems and the inevitability of a plurality of meanings existing therein, with the limits on any one perspective that this plurality implies. Finally, we have argued that only within a conversation about these meanings, which suspends arguments about reality, can important emotional truth emerge in psychoanalysis. We close the chapter with a parable illustrating the epistemological attitude of perspectival realism.

The Parable of the Blind Men and the Elephant

It was six men of Indostan
To learning much inclined,
Who went to see the Elephant
Though all of them were blind,
That each by observation
Might satisfy his mind.

The First approached the Elephant
And, happening to fall
Against his broad and sturdy side,
At once began to bawl:
"God bless me, but the Elephant
Is very like a wall!"

The Second, feeling the tusk,
Cried, "Ho! what have we here
So very round and smooth and sharp?
To me 'tis very clear
This wonder of an Elephant
Is very like a spear!"

The Third approached the animal

And, happening to take
The squirming trunk within his hands,
Thus boldly up he spake:
"I see," quoth he, "The Elephant
Is very like a snake!"

The Fourth reached out an eager hand,
And felt about the knee:
"What most the wondrous beast is like
Is very plain," quoth he;
"Tis clear enough the Elephant
Is very like a tree!"

The Fifth, who chanced to touch the ear,
Said, "Even the blindest man
Can tell what this resembles most;
Deny the fact who can:
This marvel of an elephant
Is very like a fan!"

The Sixth no sooner had begun
About the beast to grope
Than, seizing on the swinging tail
That fell within his scope,
"I see," quoth he, "the Elephant
Is very like a rope!"

And so these men of Indostan
Disputed loud and long,
Each in his own opinion
Exceeding stiff and strong.
Though each was partly in the right,
They all were in the wrong!

—**John Godfrey Saxe**

7

Worlds of Trauma

written in collaboration with Julia M. Schwartz

God is dead.
> —Friedrich Nietzsche

After the primordial phenomenon of Being-in-the-world has been shattered, the isolated subject is all that remains.
> —Martin Heidegger

In this chapter, we elaborate our conception of trauma as the shattering of an experiential world. We begin with an account of a six-year journey of understanding in which one of us strove to comprehend the profound sense of estrangement and isolation that was a central feature of his own personal experience of psychological trauma (reprinted from Stolorow, 1999).

An Autobiographical Account

When the book *Contexts of Being* (Stolorow and Atwood, 1992) was first published, an initial batch of copies was sent "hot-off-the-press" to the display table at a conference where I was a panelist. I picked up a copy and looked around excitedly for my late wife, Daphne, who would be so pleased and happy to see it. She was, of course, nowhere to be found, having died some eighteen months earlier. I had awakened one morning to find her lying dead across our bed, four weeks after her cancer had been diagnosed. I spent the remainder of that conference in 1992 remembering and grieving, consumed with feelings of horror and sorrow over what had happened to Daphne and to me.

There was a dinner at that conference for all the panelists, many of whom were my old and good friends and close colleagues. Yet, as I looked around the ballroom, they all seemed like strange and alien beings to me. Or more accurately, *I* seemed like a strange and alien being— not of this world. The others seemed so vitalized, engaged with one another in a lively manner. I, in contrast, felt deadened and broken, a shell of the man I had once been. An unbridgeable gulf seemed to open up, separating me forever from my friends and colleagues. They could never even begin to fathom my experience, I thought to myself, because we now lived in altogether different worlds.

In the years following that painful occasion, I have been trying to understand and conceptualize the dreadful sense of estrangement and isolation that seems to me to be inherent in the experience of psychological trauma. I have become aware that this sense of alienation and aloneness appears as a common theme in the trauma literature (e.g., Herman, 1992), and I have been able to hear about it from many of my patients who have experienced severe traumatization. One such young man, who had suffered multiple losses of beloved family members during his childhood and adulthood, told me that the world was divided into two groups—the normals and the traumatized ones. There was no possibility, he said, for a normal to ever grasp the experience of a traumatized one. I remembered how important it had been to me to believe that the analyst I saw after Daphne's death was also a person who had known devastating loss, and how I implored her not to say anything that could disabuse me of my belief.

How was this experiential chasm separating the traumatized person from other human beings to be understood? In the chapter on trauma in *Contexts of Being*, we had proposed that the essence of psychological trauma lay in the experience of unbearable affect. The intolerability of an affect state, we further argued, could not be explained solely, or even primarily, on the basis of the quantity or intensity of the painful feelings evoked by an injurious event. Developmentally, traumatic affect states had to be understood in terms of the relational systems in which they took form. Painful or frightening affect became traumatic, we contended, when the attunement that the child needed from the surround to assist in its tolerance, containment, modulation, and integration was profoundly absent.

In my experience, this conceptualization of developmental trauma as a relational process involving massive malattunement to painful affect has proven to be of enormous clinical value in the treatment of traumatized patients. Yet, as I began to recognize at that conference dinner, our formulation failed to distinguish between an attunement that cannot be supplied by others and an attunement that cannot be *felt* by the traumatized person, because of the profound sense of singularity built into the experience of trauma itself. A beginning comprehension of this isolating estrangement came from an unexpected source—the philosophical hermeneutics of Hans-Georg Gadamer.

Concerned as it is with the nature of understanding, philosophical hermeneutics has immediate relevance for the profound despair about having one's experience understood that lies at the heart of psychological trauma. Axiomatic for Gadamer ([1975] 1991) is the proposition that all understanding involves interpretation. Interpretation, in turn, can only be from a perspective embedded in the historical matrix of the interpreter's own traditions. Understanding, therefore, is always from a perspective whose horizons are delimited by the historicity of the interpreter's organizing principles, by the fabric of preconceptions that Gadamer calls "prejudice." Gadamer illustrates his hermeneutical philosophy by applying it to the anthropological problem of attempting to understand an alien culture in which the forms of social life, the horizons of experience, are incommensurable with those of the investigator.

At some point while studying Gadamer's work, I recalled my feeling at the conference dinner as though I were an alien to the normals around me. In Gadamer's terms, I was certain that the horizons of their experience could never encompass mine, and this conviction was the source of my alienation and solitude, of the unbridgeable gulf separating me from their understanding. It is not just that the traumatized ones and the normals live in different worlds; it is that these discrepant worlds are felt to be *essentially and ineradicably incommensurable.*

Some six years after the conference dinner I heard something in a lecture delivered by my friend George

Atwood that helped me to comprehend further the nature of this incommensurability. In the course of discussing the clinical implications of an intersubjective contextualism from which Cartesian objectivism had been expunged, Atwood offered a nonobjectivist, dialogic definition of psychotic delusions: "Delusions are ideas whose validity is not open for discussion." This definition fit well with a proposal we had made a dozen years earlier that, when a child's perceptual and emotional experiences meet with massive and consistent invalidation, then his or her belief in the reality of such experiences will remain unsteady and vulnerable to dissolution, and further, that under such predisposing circumstances delusional ideas may develop that "serve to dramatize and reify [an] endangered psychic reality . . . restoring [the] vanishing belief in its validity" (Stolorow, Brandchaft, and Atwood, 1987, p. 133). Delusional ideas were understood as a form of absolutism—a radical decontextualization serving vital restorative and defensive functions. Experiences that are insulated from dialogue cannot be challenged or invalidated.

After hearing Atwood's presentation, I began to think about the role such absolutisms unconsciously play in everyday life. When a person says to a friend, "I'll see you later," or a parent says to a child at bedtime, "I'll see you in the morning," these are statements, like delusions, whose validity is not open for discussion. Such absolutisms are the basis for a kind of naive realism and optimism that allow one to function in the world, experienced as stable and predictable. It is in the essence of psychological trauma that it shatters these absolutisms, a catastrophic loss of innocence that permanently alters one's sense of being-in-the-world. Massive deconstruction of the absolutisms of everyday life exposes the inescapable contingency of existence on a universe that is random and unpredictable and in which no safety or continuity of being can be assured. Trauma thereby exposes "the unbearable embeddedness of being" (Stolorow and Atwood, 1992, p. 22). As a result, the traumatized person cannot help but perceive aspects of existence that lie well outside the absolutized horizons of normal everydayness. It is in this sense that the worlds of traumatized persons are fundamentally incommensurable with those of others, the deep chasm in which an anguished sense of estrangement and solitude takes form.

A patient of mine who had tried to cope with a long string of traumatic violations, shocks, and losses by using dissociative processes left her young son at a pastry shop on the way to my office. As she was about to enter my building, she heard the sound of screeching tires, and in the session she was visibly terrified that her son had been struck by a car and killed. "Yes," I said, with a matter-of-factness that can only come from firsthand experience, "this is the legacy of your experiences with terrible trauma. You know that at any moment those you love can be struck down by a senseless, random event. Most people don't really know that." My patient relaxed into a state of calm and, with obvious allusion to the transference, began to muse about her lifelong yearning for a soulmate with whom she could share her experiences of trauma and thereby come to feel like less of a strange and alien being. It is here, I believe, that we find the deeper meaning of Kohut's (1984) concept of twinship. (Stolorow, 1999, pp. 464–467)

At the close of this autobiographical account, a question was posed: "If trauma can have such a devastating impact on a middle-aged man . . . how can we begin to comprehend its impact on a small child for whom the sustaining absolutisms of everyday life are just in the process of forming?" (p. 467). It is to this question that we turn here by describing a clinical case in which severe trauma occurred in the presymbolic phase of childhood. In trying to grasp this case, we hypothesize a primal absolutism, taking form in early infancy through attuned holding and handling of the child's body (Winnicott, 1965) and containment and modulation of painful affect states (Bion, 1977; Stolorow and Atwood, 1992), which we characterize as a sense of sensorimotor integrity—a presymbolic sense of one's physical being as inviolable. The case demonstrates the lifelong impact of the early shattering of sensorimotor integrity. (Alternatively, when speaking of trauma in early infancy, one might say that sensorimotor integrity was not even established at all.)

Amy, a thirty-year-old single woman, sought analytic treatment because of severe, chronic, and disabling depression, obsessions and phobias, and an inability to achieve any physical sexual intimacy. Although she longed to marry and have a child, she had never been involved in a relationship with a man. She was afraid that she might be a lesbian, although she said she had never felt sexual feelings for a woman.

In early infancy, beginning at the age of two or three months, Amy began screaming with pain while having bowel movements. As a result of a misdiagnosis, her mother had been instructed to dilate her anus digitally several times a day. When the pain persisted without improvement, her mother brought her to a specialist, and the problem was correctly diagnosed as an anal fissure and was treated appropriately. Amy herself had no recollection of these events, and her mother claimed that the digital penetrations of her child's anus occurred only a few times. According to a report from an early psychiatric consultation, however, the anal penetrations continued for several months until Amy was eight months old. Although the anal fissure healed by the time she was one year old, she engaged in painful struggles with her mother over toilet training and showed other behavioral difficulties. She was sent to her first psychiatric consultation at the age of two and one-half, because of tantrums and a refusal to speak. The consultant's report noted that when Amy refused to comply with her mother over toileting, her mother tried to insert suppositories, repeating, we believe, the early traumatic violations of the child's bodily integrity, and Amy would run away in terror. When her mother tried to make her speak, Amy would refuse stubbornly, apparently attempting thereby to restore the sense of inviolability that was being relentlessly obliterated.

Amy had few memories of her father, who clearly preferred her older brother and seemed to find her personality intolerable. When her father and brother spent time together and left Amy out, she responded by intruding on them, wreaking all manner of havoc. This intrusiveness became a hallmark of her personality in childhood. In order not to be excluded from anything, she invaded and penetrated others, much as she had been traumatically violated from an early age. Clearly, from very early on, attachment for Amy became equivalent to invasion, either invading or being invaded.

Amy's father died of lung cancer when she was seven years old. After his death, she "descended into a mire of symptoms." She became afraid of dying in her sleep and suffered from recurring stomachaches. She questioned her mother endlessly about her father's death, wanting every detail told to her over and over again. She became preoccupied with the belief that she, too, had cancer, imploring her mother to take her to the doctor to be checked for lumps. Clearly, it seems to us, her father's illness and death dramatically confirmed for Amy what she already "knew"—that her body was in constant danger of being invaded by painful, destructive, even deadly forces.

Her mother's reaction to the father's death was also very frightening for Amy, yet another intrusion into whatever tenuous feeling of security she could muster. The mother became severely depressed and made several suicidal threats and gestures, sometimes seeming to hold Amy responsible for her troubles. Amy's sense of bodily integrity was further disrupted by an early onset of puberty. It was during adolescence that an episode that Amy described as her "mental breakdown" occurred, precipitated by her mother's contracting stomach flu. Amy reacted by becoming terrified of catching her mother's illness and of throwing up. She had been phobic about vomiting since childhood, but the fears now became acute and disabling, dramatically expressing her dread of being reinvaded by her mother, both physically and emotionally.

In college, Amy excelled academically but floundered socially. After graduating, she began working in a literary agency. She had men friends, and an occasional man expressed romantic interest in her, but she never progressed beyond a single kiss.

Amy's gastrointestinal tract, the original site of trauma, continued in her adult life to be a source of conflict, pain, and dysregulation, dramatizing the extent to which her experiential world had become organized around the dread of invasion by toxic forces. By the time she had begun analysis, she had obtained multiple gastrointestinal evaluations, including radiologic and invasive procedures. She suffered from severe and alternating diarrhea and constipation and, most agonizing, acute abdominal pain and cramping. She was tormented by an overwhelming fear of, and fascination with, vomiting. She was terrified of exposure to stomach flu and would go to great lengths to protect herself from contamination, wearing a face mask when flying, using alcohol pads on her hands, and avoiding children and anyone suspected of illness. Over the years, she had banned more and more foods from her diet, believing that they were the source of her pain. She was suspicious of her mother's cooking and hygiene, fearing accidental and even intentional poisoning at her hands. Amy and her analyst understood these symptoms and phobias as expressing a fear of retraumatization—of a painful and frightening invasion of her body by deadly toxins, recapitulating her early loss of the sense of being inviolable, of sensorimotor integrity.

The impact of Amy's early trauma in obliterating her sense of bodily integrity also seemed reflected in a number of symptoms of sensorimotor dysregulation. She felt chronically cold, even in the summer, as though she could not regulate her body temperature. Songs on the radio would "get stuck" in her head. She was agitated by the movements of windshield wipers. She became distracted by activity outside her analyst's office during sessions and could concentrate only with the blinds closed. These and other difficulties were manifestations of an inability to filter and modulate visual and auditory stimulation. She also felt her motor skills to be poor. When she blew her nose, she seemed uncoordinated and childlike, grabbing several tissues at once and blowing and rubbing clumsily. Her gait and posture were disjointed, clumsy, and awkward.

The difficulties she experienced in relationships similarly reflected the central theme of vulnerability to toxic invasion, both physical and psychological. She reacted with intense aversion to people whom she experienced as pushy and controlling—to her brother, for example, who would "jam his opinions down my throat." As she, in the course of treatment, began to date more, she experienced the men as self-absorbed intruders, not interested in her ideas and only wanting to talk about themselves. Over the course of her therapy, she became able to articulate her deep and paralyzing fears of being close to a man, her revulsion at kissing, and her rage at having to "submit" to a man's advances. She found it impossible to be physically intimate with a man without these aversive feelings erupting. She would become preoccupied with men's physical imperfections, as though seeing them under a microscope—moles, pimples, facial hair, receding hairlines, and the like. She would feel suffocated by an embrace or by the smell of a man's breath. As she pushed herself toward greater physical closeness, she was barely able to tolerate her revulsion at having a man's tongue "rammed down my throat." Rather than the revulsion and anxiety being diminished by these attempts, she felt an almost allergic response, becoming hypersensitized to the experience, making it even more difficult to go on subsequent dates where more intimacy would be expected.

In the analysis, Amy rapidly developed an intense, archaic attachment to her female analyst. For example, in the third session, she confessed to making numerous calls to the analyst's office and a call to her home and to driving by the office several times. She became obsessively preoccupied with obtaining information about the analyst: where she lived, the car she drove, and other personal data. When the analyst was not forthcoming, Amy would seek out the information on her own—for example, by calling the analyst's medical school. Additionally, she became preoccupied with trying to look like her analyst, duplicating her hairstyle and wardrobe. "Do I want to become you or fuck you?" she wondered tellingly. At one point, Amy realized that being like her analyst also helped her to feel a distance from her mother.

Amy discovered the location of the analyst's home and made daily visits there to monitor what was going on. She would record the mileage on the analyst's car so that she could know of any trips the analyst took. She engaged in "stakeouts," sitting outside movie theaters, for example, for hours on end, in the hope of seeing her analyst during the weekends.

The analyst was overwhelmed by the force and intensity of Amy's preoccupation with her. More and more, it felt to the analyst like a repetition of Amy's early trauma. Now the analyst was being subjected to a painful and humiliating invasion of her personal space, as Amy had been in infancy, and Amy was taking on the role of the violator.

Amy's enactments escalated until there was an even more dramatic breach of the analyst's privacy. The analyst realized that she was living in a state of hypervigilance, monitoring her surroundings, in danger of having her personal space invaded at any time, never being able to relax fully. Her very identity was being usurped, which she found unnerving and maddening. The analyst found herself stubbornly unwilling to answer personal questions, and, just as Amy felt satisfied when she found and wore clothing similar to the analyst's or discovered something about the analyst's personal life, so the analyst found herself feeling uncomfortably but vindictively pleased when Amy could not achieve these aims. This stubborn withholding was an aspect of the analyst's personality unhappily awakened by Amy's intrusiveness.

Over time, and with supervisory consultation, the analyst was able to acknowledge the degree to which Amy's enactments had come into conflict with her own need for privacy. The analyst spelled out to Amy the ways in which she had been experiencing Amy's behavior as painful and humiliating invasions of her private space. At one point the analyst said, with considerable exasperation, that it felt like Amy was chasing her around the room trying to stick a finger up her ass. She pointed out that by continuing this behavior, Amy was jeopardizing the bond she so desperately needed. The analyst began to set strict limits on the enactments that Amy had been engaging in outside the office and to make firm decisions about what she felt comfortable disclosing to Amy when she asked questions or made requests. As they explored the meanings of her questions and of their going unanswered, there was a shift in the therapeutic relationship. Amy required less information, and, correspondingly, the analyst came to experience Amy's curiosity and questions more as interest than invasion. In retrospect, Amy benefited significantly from

the analyst's having provided a model for the firm maintenance and protection of personal boundaries, and of
attachment without violation.

Over the course of the therapy, Amy and her analyst
understood the impact of the early trauma as a frightening, painful, and obliterating invasion of Amy's body.
Consequently, physical closeness and intimacy were felt as
invasive, traumatic, and dangerously out of her control.
Amy and her analyst surmised that the mother's own guilt
and distress during those early episodes of bodily violation
made it difficult if not impossible for her to respond
empathically, to help Amy process and bear the painful
procedure and accompanying traumatic affect states.
Indeed, in subsequent years the mother tried to deny the
extent to which the trauma had even happened. Because
the trauma occurred in early infancy, prior to the capacity
for symbolization, it remained presymbolically encoded as
an "emotional memory" (Orange, 1995), outside the
horizons of verbal articulation and capable of being experienced only in the form of diffuse psychosomatic states or
behavioral enactments. Time and again, the later traumas
and difficulties in Amy's life were assimilated as repetitions
and confirmations of what had been encoded presymbolically. Many of her symptoms and phobias were also understood as manifestations of her pervasive sense that she was
in constant danger of being destructively penetrated and
invaded, and of her attempt to protect herself from such
painful attack. Amy and her analyst also eventually understood how the same emotional memory and sense of
endangerment were enacted in the therapeutic relationship, with the analyst then feeling traumatically and
painfully invaded.

As a result of the therapeutic work, Amy made considerable gains. She became able to tolerate increasing degrees of separation from the analyst. As her appearance and manner improved, partly as a result of her identifying with the analyst, and as she achieved notable success in her career, she seemed to be moving closer and closer to seeing herself as an attractive, competent, desirable woman. She was asked out on dates with increasing frequency, but still she could not tolerate much physical closeness without having an "allergic" reaction to the men.

Then tragically, while continuing to progress in the eighth year of therapy, Amy became ill with a progressive neurological disorder. Learning of this illness had an extraordinarily devastating impact on her. For her, it was the medical confirmation of her lifelong view of herself as inherently flawed, undesirable, and doomed to die alone. More important, it was a horrifying repetition of the early traumatic invasion of her body—now by toxic forces that could disable, disfigure, and literally destroy her—shattering once again her barely consolidated sense of the integrity of her physical being. Whatever progress had been made in the transformation of her self-experience seemed eradicated by the diagnosis and by the symptoms she was having. The progress she had made in feeling safe with human contact and closeness was also undone. Indeed, she even entertained a fantasy that the illness had been caused by the poisoning impact of other people in her life. In the first months after her condition was diagnosed, Amy's prognosis seemed very grim, and she and her analyst were both in a state of shock and grief. With pharmacological treatment, however, Amy's symptoms abated somewhat, and she and the analyst began the difficult task of trying to regain their equilibrium. Amy's wish to have a relationship with a man once again became prominent. She expressed frustration that so much time had passed with little improvement in her ability to have a romantic and sexual life. Even more discouraging was the recognition that in certain ways she was worse; her phobic avoidance of food, sun, cold, and germs had been greatly intensified by the impact of her medical condition. How could she hope to attract a man now that she was shackled by her illness and all its dreadful effects?

Amy and her analyst have continued to focus on the consequences of Amy's early bodily trauma and the later childhood losses and disruptions and on the retraumatizing impact of her current illness. Although Amy complained that there was nothing new in what they were discussing, she has seemed more able to take chances—with her appearance and on dates, for example. Yet the analyst cannot help but wonder how a psychoanalytic process can alter the impact of an early trauma, now devastatingly reanimated, that lives presymbolically in Amy's body. This is a question that lies at the frontier of psychoanalytic understanding. There still remains much to be learned.

8

Shattered Worlds/Psychotic States: The Experience of Personal Annihilation

Things fall apart; the centre cannot hold.
—**William Butler Yeats**

One of the most dramatic consequences of adopting a consistently phenomenological, post-Cartesian viewpoint is the opening up of the most severe ranges of psychological disorder—the so-called psychoses—to psychoanalytic understanding and treatment. This opening occurs because the experiences that characterize these psychological disturbances tend to cluster around themes of personal annihilation and the destruction of the world. Such experiences occur outside the horizon of Cartesian systems of thought, which rest upon a vision of the mind as an isolated existent that stands in relation to a stable, external reality. The Cartesian image of mind, rigidly separating an internal mental subject from an externally real object, reifies and universalizes a very specific pattern of experience, centering around an enduringly stable sense of personal selfhood that is felt as distinct and separate from a world outside. Experiences of extreme self-loss and the disintegration of the world cannot be conceptualized within such an ontology of mind, because they dissolve the very structures this ontology posits as universally constitutive of personal existence.

Some authors (Bernstein, 1983; Toulmin, 1990; Orange, 1995) have pointed to the defensive function of the Cartesian search for certainty and the associated doctrine of mind in allaying feelings of chaos, uncertainty, and trauma. Such feelings, magnified by catastrophic historical events in the era during which Descartes's ideas emerged, and strengthened as well by the losses and discontinuities of Descartes's personal development (Scharfstein, 1980; Gaukroger, 1995), perhaps in the far extreme approach the level of annihilation to which this chapter is addressed. Theories predicated on Cartesian principles that serve to avert the occurrence of such experiences also have an effect of rendering those experiences opaque to psychoanalytic understanding.

In what follows, we describe this extreme range of psychological disorder from an intersubjective, phenomenological point of view. Intersubjectivity theory, as discussed throughout this book, is a post-Cartesian psychoanalytic perspective that takes as its central focus the world of experience of the individual, understood in its own terms and without reference to an external objective reality. This world in addition is always seen in the relational context of interaction with other such worlds. The intersubjective analysis of annihilation states outlined here was significantly influenced by a number of twentieth-century psychoanalytic thinkers, including Carl Jung ([1907] 1965), Victor Tausk (1917), Paul Federn (1952), Winnicott (1958a, 1965), Ronald Laing (1959), Austin Des Lauriers

(1962), Harold Searles (1965), and Heinz Kohut (1971, 1977, 1984), who departed significantly from a Cartesian worldview even as they remained bound to the Cartesian tradition in other aspects. We begin our analysis by revisiting the classical distinction between neurosis and psychosis.

Neurosis and Psychosis

The criterion according to which the distinction between neurosis and psychosis has traditionally been made lies in an assessment of the patient's contact with objective reality. Psychosis, by definition, is a condition involving a break with reality, whereas neurosis is seen as a pathological condition in which contact with reality is preserved. Illustrating this long-standing view are Freud's well-known papers, "Neurosis and Psychosis" ([1924] 1961c) and "The Loss of Reality in Neurosis and Psychosis" ([1924] 1961b), in which he tried to delineate the similarities and differences between these broad categories of psychopathology by reference to the tripartite structural model of the mind. He argued that in both instances, the patient's difficulties ultimately arise from "the lack of fulfillment of one of those eternal uncontrollable childhood wishes that are rooted so deeply in our constitution" ([1924] 1961c, p. 187), that is, from unsatisfied id impulses. The difference between neurosis and psychosis, according to his description, lies in the way the conflict between unsatisfied instinctual desires and the forces that oppose them becomes reconciled. In the case of neurosis, "the ego remains true in its allegiance to the outer world and endeavors to subjugate the id," whereas in psychosis, the ego "allows itself to be overwhelmed by the id and [is] thus torn away from reality" ([1924] 1961c, p. 187). In a similar but more complex formulation (Freud, [1924] 1961b), neurosis and psychosis are pictured as originating from a rebellion on the part of the id against the frustrations of the outer world. The conflict is resolved in each instance in two stages:

> [The first stage is] the tearing away of the ego from reality, while [in neurosis] the second [stage] tries to make good the damage done and reestablish the relation to reality at the expense of the id . . . With psychosis, the second step is an attempt to make good the loss of reality, not, however, at the expense of a restriction laid on the id, but in another, a more lordly manner, by creating a new reality which is no longer open to objections like that which has been forsaken. (pp. 203–204)

Freud summarizes the difference by stating that "in neurosis a part of reality is avoided by a sort of flight, but in psychosis it is remodeled" (p. 204). This remodeling is a matter of a "new phantastic outer world of a psychosis [that] attempts to set itself in place of external reality" (p. 204).

The distinction between neurosis and psychosis, so understood, is predicated on a view of the mind that is quintessentially Cartesian, envisioning the person as a being—a thinking thing—that either accurately or inaccurately apprehends a surrounding external reality. The judgment as to whether the patient's experiences are in correct alignment with this objectively true world, in Freudian psychoanalysis and in traditional psychiatry generally, is left to the observing clinician, who is assumed to be in a privileged position to determine what is and is not true and real.

How are the clinical differences between neurosis and psychosis to be seen within a phenomenological, post-Cartesian framework? Does this question even have coherence in light of the fact that this very distinction rests upon Cartesian foundations? A focus on experience leads analysts away from judgments as to the veracity of what is perceived and believed and toward an assessment of personal realities and subjective worlds in their own terms, without any reference to an external standard of the real. While recognizing that such a revised approach necessarily undercuts the basis for any sharp dichotomy between these psychopathological groupings and that clinicians are more likely to find themselves working with some sort of continuum defined by various dimensions of subjectivity, we can give a preliminary answer that the so-called psychoses do show experiences not appearing with equal salience in the range of the diagnostically neurotic and normal. These experiences, as noted earlier, center around a theme of personal annihilation, a subject that we will now consider in greater detail.

The Experience of Personal Annihilation

An aura of impenetrability has always surrounded the psychoses, which have seemed far removed from ordinary experience and therefore extremely difficult or even impossible to reach empathically. This felt difficulty is indeed inherent in the very definition of these conditions, insofar as their essential feature is regarded as being a departure from the putatively true and real world a normal person inhabits. The obstacles to establishing empathy for the subjective states appearing in this extreme range of psychological disorder, however, are in our view not solely due to the experiences involved being at some distant remove from the average, normal life of a human being. A very powerful impediment arises from an altogether different source, namely, the assumptions of the observing clinician about the nature of experience itself and ultimately about the nature of a person. When one is regarded as possessing a mind, and this mind in turn is conceived as having an interior that is occupied by conscious (and perhaps unconscious) psychic contents, a structure is being imposed that sharply delineates the boundaries of one's personhood in respect to an objectively real outer world. As we have noted, such a picture dichotomizes the subjective field into an inside and an outside, reifies and rigidifies the distinction between them, and envisions the resulting structure as constitutive of human existence in general.

Once we understand how the Cartesian view of the person reifies and universalizes this very specific pattern of experience, we can also see why the subjective states that appear so prominently in the psychoses could never be adequately encompassed by a conceptual system resting on Cartesian premises. These states include experiences of the dissolution of boundaries demarcating I and not-I, of the fragmentation and dispersal of one's very identity, and of the disintegration of reality itself. A phenomenological framework, by contrast, is unencumbered by objectifying images of mind, psyche, or psychical apparatus and is therefore free to study experience without evaluating it for its veridicality with respect to a presumed external reality.

The exploration of annihilation states accordingly presents no special philosophical difficulty, for we are concerned then only with the person and his or her world, in whatever state they may present themselves.

In the study of psychological annihilation, one may focus on self-experience or, more broadly, on world experience, where the former is seen as a central area included within the latter. Experiences of selfhood and worldhood are inextricably bound up with one another, in that any dramatic change in the one necessarily entails corresponding changes in the other. Self-dissolution, for example, is not a subjective event that could leave the world of the individual otherwise intact, with the selfhood of the person somehow subtracted out. The experience of self-loss means the loss of an enduring center in relation to which the totality of the individual's experiences are organized. The dissolution of one's selfhood thus produces an inevitable disintegrating effect on the person's experience in general and results ultimately in the loss of coherence of the world itself. Likewise, the breakup of the unity of the world means the loss of a stable reality in relation to which the sense of self is defined and sustained, and an experience of self-fragmentation inevitably follows in its wake. World disintegration and self-dissolution are thus inseparable aspects of a single process, two faces of the same psychological catastrophe.

The experience of annihilation lies at the heart of the psychoses, and this is often expressed directly in statements to the effect that the person is dead or dying, that he or she has no self, does not exist, or is absent rather than present. Those who have experienced annihilation also frequently say that the world is not real, that it has broken apart into pieces, and even that it is coming to an end. Sometimes the destruction of one's personal reality appears in an experience of falling forever, of spinning out of control, of shrinking endlessly and disappearing, or of being swallowed up into the environmental surround. More commonly, however, reparative and restorative efforts to reestablish a sense of existing predominate in the clinical picture, and these efforts appear in a wide variety of forms. A sense of being or becoming unreal, for example, gives rise to a preoccupation with one's mirror reflection, as if sustained attention to the visual outline of one's bodily being could compensate for a vanishing sense of personal selfhood. The experience of a deadness at the core of one's existence leads to a search for a counteracting sense of aliveness, provided by the intensity of sensation in self-inflicted pain, in bizarre sexuality, or in thrilling, death-defying adventures. The dissolving of bodily boundaries and a terrifying feeling of melting into one's surroundings occasions the wearing of multiple sets of clothing, one on top of the next, expressing an attempt to reestablish and protect a devastated sense of bounded self-integrity. A breakup in the felt continuity of personal identity over time brings about an obsession with recalling and mentally reliving large numbers of events from the recent and remote past, the calling up of the various events embodying an effort to bring the temporally separated fragments of history together into a single whole. An experience of the disintegration of reality itself, of the falling apart of the world into a jumble of unconnected perceptions and meaningless happenings, gives way to delusions of reference in which the isolated elements are woven back together and given a sinister, directly personal significance. Small changes in the appearance of familiar people seem to indicate global changes and breaches of identity, heralding the fragmentation of the world's stability into temporal chaos, and these breaks in continuity are repaired and smoothed over by the delusional idea that these people have somehow been replaced by nefarious impostors. In each of these instances, a countervailing effort to reintegrate a fragmenting world and restore a sense of continuous and coherent being is most salient, while the underlying annihilation state recedes into the background.

In other cases, the annihilation itself is foregrounded, often in vividly concrete symbols, so that images of personal destruction pervade and dominate the individual's experience. Here the extremes to which the concretization is carried assist in maintaining the state of one's dissolving selfhood in focal awareness. The image of being poisoned by deadly chemicals or invisible gases, for example, concretely portrays a sense of being infiltrated and then killed off by the impinging, intrusive impacts of the social surround. Picturing a distant machine that sends influencing rays into one's mind and body likewise articulates an experience of the loss of agency[1] and of falling under the obliterating control of an alien agenda. Murdering assassins or conspiring government agents are imagined, and these figures concretize the threat of psychological obliteration in the face of irresistible pressures from emotionally significant others. A takeover of one's brain by a supernatural entity is suddenly felt to occur,

---

[1] Terms such as *agency, authenticity, cohesion,* and so on are used here in an exclusively phenomenological sense, referring to dimensions of self-experience along which annihilation states typically take form (Orange, Atwood, and Stolorow, 1997, chap. 4).

symbolizing an overpowering invalidation and usurpation of one's subjectivity.

Sometimes the imagery of annihilation is intermixed with or even supplanted by what appear to be grandiose or highly idealized visions of oneself or others. These latter images express efforts to resurrect all those parts of one's selfhood and world that have become subject to shattering and erasure. The concepts of grandiosity and idealization are, however, problematic when understood in the context of the phenomenology of personal annihilation. Identifying a particular experience as idealized or grandiose involves a judgment and a standard defining what is and is not reasonable for a person to believe. Grandiosity means appropriating to oneself a significance, power, and perfection one actually does not possess. Idealization, as this term is traditionally employed, means correspondingly exaggerating the significance and perfection of some emotionally important other. In the context of personal annihilation, however, it cannot be said that so-called idealization and grandiosity appropriate or exaggerate anything. What appears, from an external point of reference, to be an outrageous exaggeration may, subjectively regarded, be understood as accentuating the sense that one exists, that one possesses agency and subjectivity, that one's experiences belong to no one other than oneself, and that one's personal world has coherence and is enduringly real. A delusional claim to be the owner of the world, for example, may contain at its core a dissolving sense of one's perceptions and thoughts being one's own. Seemingly extravagant assertions of personal achievement and capability may crystallize and intensify an otherwise threatened experience of agency and autonomy. Visions of descending from a royal lineage or of being a specially chosen child of God accentuate and protect a disappearing sense of connection to a world-sustaining other. The idea that one has penetrated the ultimate secret of the cosmos, the key to understanding the interrelationships of all existing things, enshrines and preserves the integrity of one's personal world in the face of a threat of its total disintegration. In each of these last four examples, the problematic issue is not that unrealistic grandiose or idealized qualities are being ascribed to oneself or others; it is rather that the individual's personal universe has come under assault and is in danger of annihilation. Let us turn now to the intersubjective contexts in which the experiences we have been describing take form.

The Intersubjective Context of Annihilation

In a previous work (Orange, Atwood, and Stolorow, 1997), we said that the experience of personal annihilation reflects an intersubjective catastrophe in which psychologically sustaining relations to others have broken down at their most fundamental level. What does this breakdown entail? It consists in the loss of affirming, validating connections to others and the shattering of the subjective world by impingement and usurpation. Although the concrete events and life circumstances playing a role in the origin of annihilation states are highly varied, they have in common an effect of undermining one's sense of existing and of being real in its most basic aspects, including the experience of oneself as an active agent and subject, as possessing an identity that is coherent and felt as authentically one's own, as having a boundary delineating and delimiting I and not-I, and as being continuous in time and over history.

Viewing psychological annihilation in the context of an intersubjective field means that this experience is interpreted as occurring within a living system of mutual influence. The visible manifestations of the experience are therefore not seen to emanate from a pathological condition localized solely within the patient; nor, however, are they regarded simply as reactions to a primary victimization at the hands of others. Such unilateral conceptions, emphasizing an exclusive determination either from the side of the patient or from the side of the human environment, fail to take into account the complex transactional process occurring between the two. Sometimes people undergoing the experiences described here are viewed as carrying a special vulnerability or even a predisposition that is then seen as a determinative factor in the genesis of personal annihilation. The problem with such an idea is that it represents a return to Cartesian and objectivist thinking, within which factors somehow located "inside" an individual—in his or her mind or brain—become operative causes in the unfolding of subjective states. We then have a picture of an isolated mind, containing predisposing sensitivities and vulnerabilities, that collapses in the face of objective external pressures of some kind. In an intersubjective framework of understanding there are no fully isolable vulnerabilities that exist inside anyone, because what appears or does not appear as a vulnerability only materializes within specific intersubjective fields.

Imagine a patient who feels she is not present, does not exist, and has no self. Imagine further that a clinician not familiar with such states asks her, "How are you today?" The use of the second-person pronoun "you" implies to the patient a degree of existence she does not experience, and a gulf of misunderstanding and invalidation opens up between her and the questioner. Perhaps the patient gives the answer, "A billion light years," expressing how far away she feels from the questioner in view of the naive assumption having been made that there is a "you" to whom the inquiry would be intelligible, a "you" who could report on how it feels at the time." Perhaps the patient also experiences an invasion and usurpation by the questioner's unfounded assumptions, and she begins to speak of a machine sending rays into the center of her brain, in order to give this deepening annihilation experience form and substance. From the standpoint of the questioner, one who takes a Cartesian view of things, the patient's replies are utterly incomprehensible. The question, after all, has been appropriate and clearly phrased, and the answers coming back are without apparent connection to all that is true and real. The patient is at most a few feet rather than a billion light years away, and there is no machine in the world that can perform as the patient has now begun to claim. Clearly, the questioner thinks, this patient's sensitivities and vulnerabilities are such that the slightest human interaction triggers bizarre reactions stemming from pathological processes taking place inside the patient's mind or body. A reciprocally reinforcing intersubjective disjunction has thus arisen in which the questioner ascribes defects to the patient's mind/brain even as the patient experiences her mind/brain as being penetrated and inhabited by a foreign influence.

Now imagine a second clinician who speaks to the patient differently, who finds a way to acknowledge her sense of nonbeing and who understands as well the patient's readiness to surrender herself to whatever is attributed to her. He speaks to the patient in the third person, conveys his knowledge of how terrible it is not to exist, and in a variety of highly concrete ways lets the patient know she is not alone in the catastrophe that is the ongoing situation of her life. The patient, surprised by this different approach, actually begins to feel understood and, paradoxically, begins also to feel a flickering of her own existence, moments of directly sensed being alternating with the continuing feeling of nonexistence or nonbeing. These moments of being, occurring because of the validating experience of being seen and acknowledged, have a painful aliveness about them, dramatically contrasting with the numbness and deadness accompanying the sense of nonexistence. Perhaps the patient, after a period, says she has been stung by a swarm of bees, concretizing the sporadically recurring moments of aliveness as they alternate with episodes of the familiar deadness and nonbeing. Let us imagine further that this second clinician perceives the metaphor of this transitory delusion as well and finds ways to address the ambivalent experience the patient is having of coming back to life. Her sense of existing thus becomes strengthened again by the incomparable power of human recognition. The patient's readiness to surrender to others' attributions and definitions, itself embedded in a complex, lifelong history of intersubjective transactions, is not engaged in the foreground of this second interaction and therefore does not appear as an operative defect or vulnerability in the experiences that unfold. This is because the intersubjective field in this instance is characterized on the one side by gradually developing understanding and on the other by a predominance of validation and an increasing sense of being.

In the example just cited, we see how a clinician operating on Cartesian assumptions is not in a position to understand experiences of nonbeing. To such an observer, it is simply not true that the patient does not exist, it is not true that she is absent, and her claims about penetrating rays from influencing machines appear extravagantly delusional. Any reaction on the part of the clinician communicating this view, of course, intensifies the patient's experience of invalidation and annihilation, giving rise to a spiraling of disjunctive worlds in which the patient elaborates ever more concretized images of her obliteration and the clinician becomes ever more appalled by the spectacle of madness unfolding before his eyes. The patient's so-called delusions, in the context of this vicious spiral, emerge as expressions of subjectivity under siege, products of a war of the worlds constituted by mutual misunderstanding and mutual invalidation.

In order to further define and illustrate the context of personal annihilation, let us consider another patient, a young Catholic woman who for years had been preoccupied with visions of herself as having a special connection to God. In vivid hallucinations and elaborate delusions, she experienced a oneness with God the Father and God the Son, variously identifying with the Holy Virgin, the Holy Ghost, and Jesus Christ himself. Claiming at times to have undergone sexual union with Jesus, to have physically flown to Rome to be held in the arms of the pope, and to be channeling God's healing peace-making powers to the entire human race, the patient harbored ideas and beliefs that made it impossible for those around her to relate their own experiences to hers in meaningful dialogue. Accordingly, the patient was said to have lost contact with the real and to be psychotic. Phenomenologically, of course, no such judgment or diagnosis occurs, as one seeks instead to understand the patient in her own subjective terms, exploring the history of events that could make her situation humanly intelligible. This inquiry disclosed a pivotal incident in the patient's middle childhood years, the sudden suicide of her beloved father following devastating personal disappointments and failures in his professional life. It was discovered as well that the death was covered over by the family, falsely redefined as having been accidental, and then hidden away behind a wall of impenetrable silence. The affairs of the family thus continued as though the father's suicide had never occurred, so little being said of him that he was relegated to the effective status of someone who had never been. It was the family's turning away from the father's death and life that was the context of a gradually deepening sense of inner deadness and isolation in the patient in the years that followed. This was also the setting for her first ruminations on the figure of Jesus Christ and a special place she imagined for herself in the Holy Trinity. Over a period of more than a decade, secret religious thoughts about her relation to God gradually blossomed into full-fledged delusional realities, finally bursting forth in the family with great violence and precipitating the first of many psychiatric hospitalizations. Central in the patient's expressions at this time were loud, imperious demands that she immediately be united with Jesus, who she believed had been miraculously reincarnated in a church-affiliated counselor she had once known and depended on for a brief period.

The bond to the father, something that centrally sustained this patient as a young girl, had not only been lost when he died; his death occurred as an intentional suicide, which was unthinkable if, as she had believed during her early years, he actually loved her. Her unbearable experience of having been deserted by him, however, had itself been suppressed by the family's denial, so that the reality of all she had known with him when he was alive and of all she had felt upon losing him when he killed himself was undercut and nullified, eventually undermining her very selfhood as the feelings of deadness expanded and deepened.

How is one to understand this patient's seemingly fantastic religious claims and demands, in view of this context of abandonment and personal devastation? The Cartesian analyst, following Freud, inevitably focuses on the wide disparity between the patient's beliefs and the purportedly objective truth of her life situation, perceiving a deficiency in reality testing, a break with the objectively real and the setting up of an idealized alternative in its place. The streaming religious fantasies and delusions, from such a viewpoint, appear as wish-fulfilling substitutes for the lost connection to the father, and the patient's disturbance seems to consist precisely in her immersion in these fantasies at the expense of attention to her actual, painfully sad situation. An intersubjective analysis, by contrast, focuses on how the patient's so-called delusions protect and preserve a shattered world, how they reinstate a personal reality that has been substantially annihilated, how they embody an effort to resurrect a world-sustaining tie in the midst of an experience of complete obliteration. Far from expressing a flight from painful reality, according to this post-Cartesian view, she is understood to have used the symbols of her faith to encapsulate a remnant of the destroyed bond to her father and thereby to maintain a hold on all that was most real in her experience of herself and her world. The patient's demands to be united with Jesus Christ, urgently and aggressively reiterated in the early course of her treatment, were thus cries for the world-preserving connection upon which her very existence depended.

Viewing a person such as this as delusional highlights the disparity between her experiences and beliefs and the conditions of supposedly external reality. From this perspective, a goal inevitably materializes to bring the patient's ideas into conformity with all that is generally agreed upon as real and true. These normative beliefs have no place for special linkages to Jesus Christ and unassisted flights to Rome, such ideas being seen as pathological fantasies that need to be interpreted and relinquished or suppressed. What, one may ask, is the effect on the patient of being seen and treated in this way? Such a view inevitably communicates a message that the patient's most urgently felt desires are misguided and that her sole remaining hopes for restoring herself and her reality are without foundation. This message repeats and reinforces the emotional abandonment and invalidation she experienced at the hands of her father and her family, and its effect is to accelerate the delusional process as the patient seeks her own survival in ever more concrete, vividly dramatized ways. A vicious spiral has thus again sprung into being, in which disjunctive worlds war with one another in unending cycles of misunderstanding and reciprocal invalidation.

An analyst who understands the meaning of this patient's entreaties, by contrast, comes to her with no agenda to realign the content of her experiences; the analyst's purpose is rather to introduce a new element into her devastated life, one around which she can refind the felt core of her existence. This element will be embodied in her experience of both the analyst and the analyst's understanding, something emotionally impactful and powerful, calming and reassuring in its effect. This analyst will establish a personal presence, at first physically in space and time, by regularly appearing and reappearing, and by engaging the patient's attention through concrete, simple interactions of various kinds. When eventually the full force of her delusional efforts to salvage herself and her world become directed toward the analyst, as inevitably they will, and she pressures the analyst to reunite her with the man she believes to be Jesus Christ, the analyst will respond gently but definitively by telling her that there is only one person in the world she should be concerned about seeing and that the analyst is that person. The analyst will explain further that there are to be no meetings with anyone except for those that they have with each other, for it is in their work together that she will become well again and return home to be with those who love her. In all of these interventions, the analyst is guided by an understanding that it is the analyst who must become the inheritor of the patient's strivings and that the therapeutic relationship is the central battleground on which her psychological survival is to be worked out. How does she respond to all of these things? The delusional process, far from being exacerbated, actually begins to recede as the analyst is established as someone in relation to whom she can recover a sense of herself and of the reality of her destroyed world. At first, her dependence is extreme, and she even intimates that her newfound therapist might indeed have some special status with respect to God Almighty. Such expressions are understood as reflecting the power of the bond that is forming, a bond that undergirds a shattered universe in the process of being reassembled. The analyst accordingly gives no response to such attributions on the level of their literal content and is occupied instead with reinforcing the developing connection she has begun to experience between them. Each step in the solidification of their tie is accompanied by a further stabilization of her world and a continuing decentralizing of her religious images as their function passes over to the therapeutic relationship. In the early stages of this healing process, any disturbance in the tie that has been evolving produces extreme reactions of terror of abandonment and sometimes also a resurgence of the religious fantasies. As the threatened tie is reinstated in each instance, the terror disappears and the religious imagery recedes. In this way, the conditions are gradually established within which her experiences of abandonment, betrayal, and invalidation can begin to be addressed and healed on a lasting foundation.

Once a post-Cartesian attitude toward psychosis is adopted, as the two cases just described illustrate, new understandings crystallize, and previously unseen opportunities for therapeutic intervention appear. In pursuing the implications of this shift in perspective, we discuss two other important issues in clinical psychoanalysis to which an understanding of annihilation states is centrally relevant: the problem of mania and the nature of psychological trauma in its most extreme forms.

The Manic Protest

Manic states of mind are traditionally defined in terms of various departures of the individual's mood, thinking, and behavior from a preestablished standard of normality. Among the diagnostic signs used to identify this psychological state are such features as unrealistic euphoria; racing thoughts; extravagant, often grandiose plans and projects; hypersexuality; and extreme irritability and insensitivity to the needs and feelings of others. The application of these criteria within a Cartesian framework, invoking norms of health that are externally derived, inevitably obstructs the exploration of mania in terms of the patient's own world of experience. Psychoanalytic views of mania as a disorder of mood arising out of exclusively intrapsychic dynamics additionally leave out of consideration the relational context in which this subjective state is embedded. Two questions may accordingly be posed when a consistently post-Cartesian approach to this problem is taken. First, what are the features of mania when it is examined from a viewpoint seeking to approximate how it is experienced? Second, what is the configuration of the intersubjective field that is typically associated with the occurrence of the manic state? We approach these questions, guided by the seminal insights of Bernard Brandchaft ([1993] 1994), by briefly reviewing some experiences recounted in two autobiographical descriptions of this phenomenon: Patty Duke's *A Brilliant Madness* (Duke and Hochman, 1992) and Kay Jamison's *An Unquiet Mind* (1995).

During one of several manic episodes Duke experienced during her early adult years, a compelling delusion appeared that agents of foreign governments had infiltrated the White House. These infiltrators, she believed, were gradually assuming command of American policy. It was her mission to travel across the country and personally rescue the nation by rooting out the invaders and restoring the operations of government to American officials. A failed effort to actually carry out this mission was followed up by an episode of very severe depression. What light may be thrown upon the nature of the manic experience and its context by studying a delusion such as this one? We suggest that Duke's vision of foreign agents intruding into the decisions of American policy concretizes the psychological usurpation accompanying a surrender to others' interests and agendas in defining her identity and governing her own life course. The overriding fact of her life history relevant in this connection is that she was raised, in highly abusive and exploitative circumstances, as a creature of the entertainment industry. Delivered over to television agents and producers as a young girl, she grew up in a world that was never truly her own, becoming a nationally acclaimed star, but at the price of a stolen childhood. An understanding of the extent of her emotional captivity helps us to identify a central feature of the meaning of mania within her personal life situation. Her manic states contained at their core an attempted freeing, a breaking out or breaking away from external determinations of the content of her identity and the direction of her life. This freeing, which Brandchaft ([1993] 1994) has described as a "transient shedding of an enslaving tie" (p. 72), is of course only one side of a binary pattern, with the other side being that of surrender of oneself and one's life to the defining power of alien agendas. The dark alternative to mania, as Duke's delusional images of the plight of

American government symbolically illustrate, is continuing subjection to the ruling power of others' invasive definitions of who one is and how one must live.

It is interesting to us that *A Brilliant Madness* is actually coauthored by a science journalist, who wrote several chapters of the book chronicling Duke's history from the standpoint of biological psychiatry. These chapters, tracing the unfolding course of a physically based illness, are interposed between those sections authored by Duke, which tell the story of her life as she experienced it, from her own point of view. If we view the book as a whole as a record of the journey of Patty Duke's soul, we then become witness to how a set of wholly external determinations, like the imagined infiltrators in the White House, has taken up residence inside the structure of her narrative about herself. The autobiography of her madness thus cyclically mirrors the inner pattern of the madness itself, oscillating back and forth between a position of accommodative surrender to external authority and a position of self-expression and attempted self-liberation.

A parallel alternation between contrasting, experientially incompatible perspectives occurs in Jamison's *An Unquiet Mind*. Although this book has only a single author, two different voices are discernible in the flow of its descriptions. One voice is allied with medical authority, affirming again and again the biological underpinnings of the manic-depressive illness from which the author is said to suffer. This voice describes the events of Jamison's life as the unfolding manifestations of an organic disease. The other voice gives repeated expression to a love for the intensity of experience in her cycling mood states and only very reluctantly gives assent to her medical diagnosis and to the stabilizing drugs prescribed by her doctors. Among the many incidents recounted in this story of madness, one involves a vivid hallucination symbolically encoding important aspects of Jamison's history. She tells how one evening, following an extended period of frenetic activity and growing confusion, she suddenly felt a strange light at the back of her eyes and saw an enormous black centrifuge somehow inside her own head. Then a figure dressed in a flowing white evening gown and long white gloves approached the centrifuge with a vase-size glass tube of blood. Recognizing this figure as herself, she also saw with horror that blood covered the evening gown and gloves. The bloody figure placed the glass tube into the centrifuge and turned the machine on. Paralyzed by fear, she watched and listened as the machine spun faster and faster, and the clanking of the glass tube against the metal grew louder and louder. Finally the centrifuge burst, splintering into a thousand separate pieces. Blood was everywhere, covering everything, extending even into the sky.

How are we to understand this hallucination, and what does it tell us about Jamison's mania? The blood contained in the glass tube may be seen as a symbol of her inner vitality, bottled up within a role identity based on compliance with the conditions of her upbringing. This identity, expressed in the image of the figure in an evening gown, materializes what was expected from a young woman in the traditional military world of Jamison's childhood. As the child of an air force officer, she was expected to learn the "fine points of manners, dancing, white gloves, and other unrealities of life" (1995, p. 27), and within the setting of those expectations there was little room for the intense, mercurial girl she also describes herself as having been. The vision of the blood being sub-jected to the enormous pressures of the centrifuge gives form to the crushing effect on Jamison's self-experience of the roles she felt required to fulfill. When the centrifuge explodes, these roles are disintegrated, and a kind of free-ing of the formerly imprisoned life-spirit takes place. But this is a freeing into structureless chaos, negating the orderly, patterned world to which she had accommodated herself but containing nothing organized to take its place.

The manic state, seen from a post-Cartesian intersub-jective viewpoint, is not to be pictured solely as a defense against depression and cannot be explained as an outcome of exclusively intrapsychic transformations (Klein, [1934] 1950a; Winnicott, [1935] 1958b). A pervasively impor-tant meaning of mania is that it may express a kind of protest against annihilating accommodation to agendas and roles that are not authentically the person's own.[2] It thus provides a transitory restoration of a sense of agency and authenticity, by disrupting the "borrowed cohesion" (Brandchaft, [1993] 1994) of an identity based in com-pliance with others' agendas.

The reason this restoration can only be transitory and is always so destructive is that the manic protest is a burst-ing of familiar patterns but in the absence of any psycho-logical organization that can constitute an alternative. The classic diagnostic signs defining the manic state can thus

---

[2] This formulation is compatible with Frieda Fromm-Reichman's (1954) generalization, interpersonally rather than intersubjectively conceptualized, that the families of origin of so-called manic-depres-sive patients tend to be ones in which the child comes to serve the needs and purposes of others and is not treated as a fully separate and distinct person in his or her own right.

be understood as manifestations of this active breaking out of a surrendered life into chaotic freedom.

Manias spring into being around faint images and intuitions that are rooted in lost possibilities of authenticity, and the world that seems briefly to materialize in the manic state is accordingly charged with thrilling excitement and euphoria. Suddenly anything seems possible because a new universe of freedom has opened up, opportunities for creative self-expression abound, and for perhaps the first time in life the person has the exhilarating feeling of knowing who he or she is. In the extreme, every limit on thought and action dissolves, and chaos reigns in all the spheres of the person's existence. Finally and inevitably, the new world begins to collapse, for there is nothing and no one to sustain it, and it has no underlying organization that has ever been consolidated. At this point a crushing depression often ensues, as the old identity begins to reassert itself, and the old patterns of accommodation become reinstated (Brandchaft, [1993] 1994). The newfound freedom evaporates, the dreams of a glorious personal destiny fade away, and the briefly intensified feelings of efficacy and agency are supplanted by a deadening, annihilating inertia.

The experience of mania, like any subjective state, cannot be fully understood apart from the intersubjective context in which it appears. Efforts to "explain" this state of mind by attributing it to exclusively internal factors omit the constitutive role of the intersubjective field and risk falling into an oversimplifying reductionism. Let us turn now to a second important problem in clinical psychoanalysis: the relationship between extreme trauma and experiences of personal annihilation.

Trauma and Annihilation

Why does one person respond to trauma with a successful act of dissociation, leaving the organization of his or her world otherwise relatively intact, whereas another reacts with an experience of self- and world dissolution? Traditional psychoanalytic views tend to answer this question with concepts such as that of ego strength, appealing to a factor of intrinsic resilience existing inside the isolated mind of the individual. One is driven to this kind of an explanation as long as trauma is conceived crudely and externally, for one is then envisioning different minds responding differently to the same objective occurrences.

A post-Cartesian psychoanalytic theory, while not denying the existence of an individual's strengths, recognizes that anyone's resources only come into play within specific intersubjective fields. In addition, the nature of trauma itself is understood to vary as a partial function of the relational and historical context in which it occurs (Stolorow and Atwood, 1992). The trauma experience that leads to annihilation, embedded in its own distinctive context, is likely to differ markedly from the one in which a dissociation takes place. What is the nature of this difference? We seek an answer to this question by again turning to a clinical story, that of a young woman whose life included a long-standing pattern of dissociation of very extreme trauma and also, during her late teen years, the breakdown of this dissociation and the appearance of annihilation experiences.

The patient to be discussed was eighteen years old when she had her first psychological crisis involving a sense of personal annihilation. This crisis was ushered in by a persistent auditory hallucination that began one afternoon when she had run out of money and had no way of getting back to her parents' home. She called her mother to ask for a ride and was calmly and cheerfully told that she was perfectly capable of finding a way home on her own. She was very depressed because of a variety of extremely difficult circumstances in her life at the time, and her mother's response was disheartening and confusing. She did not think she was able to find her way anywhere and certainly felt unable to make the thirty-mile journey to her home by herself. Yet her mother had been so positive and encouraging in telling her to be self-reliant. She stood in the phone booth from which she had made the call, awash in confusing impressions from the conversation, and suddenly she heard a voice speaking: "You see . . . you're blind . . . you see . . . you're blind . . . you see . . . you're blind . . . " Again and again the voice intoned these words, frightening her and confusing her further. She did not know who was speaking, and the meaning of the things being said felt strange and seemed to shift around as she listened. The statements contradicted each other, in that the first statement said she could see, and the second one said she could not. With this confusion still unresolved, a second hearing of the voice occurred, in which it seemed to be explaining to her that she indeed could see nothing, that she was in fact blind. But if she were blind and therefore could see absolutely nothing, she wondered, how could she be expected to see that she was blind? She thought the voice was now telling her to see that she could not see anything, but she was unable to understand what this could mean. Finally the words themselves dissolved, and everything, including her own body, began to lose solidity and appear unreal. After wandering around in a disoriented state for several hours, she was picked up by the police and taken to a psychiatric hospital. Her records from that day describe her as having been in a floridly psychotic state.

There were three circumstances affecting this young woman at the time of this first breakdown. The first was that she had graduated from high school and had entered a large university in which she did not know anyone. The months preceding her crisis had been spent in growing alienation and aloneness, starkly contrasting with her earlier school experiences. During her high-school and middle-school years, she had an abundance of friends and good teachers, and she had immersed herself in enjoyable extracurricular activities. Now, however, she was in unfamiliar territory, taking classes in which she had no interest and spending long hours alone in her college dormitory room. The only break in this isolation was a series of brief sexual encounters with various young men she met, none of whom showed any inclination to become more lastingly involved with her. The second disturbing situation was that she had learned her mother was suffering from ovarian cancer that had already begun to metastasize. Recognizing that her mother could only live a year or less, she foresaw her death as the end of the normal world and normal life in which she had always tried to believe. Some of her feelings about this appeared to be symbolized in a nightmare she had at the time, involving a huge mound of earth swelling and growing menacingly in the backyard of her childhood home. She pictured the mound as a developing grave for her mother. The third overwhelming circumstance of this disastrous time involved a car accident in which the patient received a severe concussion and a knee injury that resulted in several weeks of excruciating pain. Her injured body, previously intact and reliable, had now become the site of great suffering and the source of an unprecedented sense of physical vulnerability.

The patient's catastrophic reaction to her mother's invalidating response to her request for help surely was not independent of the stressful, overpowering situations just described. How can we understand the impact of these various traumatic circumstances in contributing to her eventual experience of annihilation? The answer to this question must be sought in the patient's life history.

Until the moment of her crisis and subsequent hospitalization, she had, to outward appearances anyway, been functioning at a very high level. She had maintained an A average throughout her school years, had many lasting friendships, and was regarded as a happy person by everyone who knew her. Her family also appeared completely normal to the outside world, keeping a well-trimmed lawn, regularly attending church and participating in the PTA, and making ongoing contributions to community organizations. There was, however, a hidden madness in the family, in that the patient had been subject to secret sexual abuse by her father throughout her entire childhood. Commencing at the age of two, she had provided oral sexual gratification to her father two or more times each week. His visits to her bedroom always occurred in the middle of the night, when all the other family members were sleeping. He was very gentle with her during these encounters, awakening her with such words as, "Okay, honey, it's our special time again," and then inserting his penis into her mouth and slowly bringing himself to erection and eventual orgasm. Then he would tuck her back into bed and quietly leave. Only once did the patient say anything to anyone about the nocturnal visits, when at the age of six she described her father's actions to a schoolmate. At that time she had imagined that all fathers performed similar rituals with their daughters, and she was surprised by her friend's shock and horror. The friend told her own mother, who in turn called the patient's mother with the story. Terribly distraught, the mother phoned her family doctor and reported the whole incident. She was enormously reassured when the doctor explained that six-year-old girls commonly invent such stories as an expression of their early sexual development. Later on that same day, the mother forcefully informed the patient that she would be severely punished if she continued to make up such lies. The father, too, took his daughter aside the next day, telling her that it would be best for her to be silent regarding their special relationship. He added that people were generally not ready to understand and accept such things, but that eventually the world would change, and fathers and daughters everywhere would be having their "special times." In the royal houses of ancient Egypt and Greece, according to him, parents and children all participated in these acts of love, and the glorious achievements of these societies long ago were in part due to such practices. He continued that he and she were in fact forerunners of a new age in which the ancient ways would be revived and the world as a whole would be renewed. In the meantime, however, it would be best if she kept these matters to herself. She promised never to say anything more to anyone, and the abuse continued without interruption until the patient was thirteen years old, when a relative of the family walked in on the father having anal intercourse with the patient's younger brother.

How did the patient survive these conditions? She did so by cordoning off the nighttime experiences with her father from life during the day. During daylight hours, she never thought about what was occurring after dark, throwing herself instead into the normality of life at school and with her friends. Her father during the day was himself entirely different, appearing to be a caring, dedicated family man, and her mother acted throughout as a devoted homemaker. Politically conservative in orientation, the parents worked to instill self-reliance and righteous virtue in their children, often lecturing them over dinner on the importance of moral values and ethical conduct. On a number of occasions, the father even gave guidance to his daughter as to what to do when young men she would meet later in her life tried to draw her into sexual situations for which she was unready. Meanwhile, the night visits continued, as if on a different plane of reality, sharply dissociated from the experiences making up the very normal life of the day. The patient surrendered to her father during the secret encounters, complying with his gentle intrusions, and each day when she woke up in the morning, it was as if nothing at all had occurred the night before. She was, however, haunted by recurring nightmares throughout the period of the abuse, dreams vividly depicting her psychological situation in the family.

In one of these dreams, which she reported as having occurred dozens of times during her early and middle childhood years, she stood alone on the brightly illuminated linoleum floor of her family's kitchen. She noticed the presence on the floor of numerous tiny dark spots or dots, each no larger than a period. She then also saw that above each spot there was nothing, as if a tiny column of invisible disintegrating power emanated upward from the floor. Any object extending spatially over the floor had holes in it that were precisely the size of the spots directly beneath. As she stared at the strange dots of darkness, she noticed them changing and slowly becoming enlarged. As the spots grew, the holes in objects above them also grew, and soon whole sectors of the kitchen lighting, cupboards, and ceiling were beginning to disappear. Inasmuch as she was herself standing on that same floor, the expanding spots threatened her as well, and the dream always ended as she fearfully moved and danced around the expanding darkness, trying always to stay in the light. The imagery of darkness and light in this dream appeared to connect with the conditions of the split daylight and nighttime worlds of the patient's childhood. During the day, everything was as it should be: Her mother and father acted like and actually were concerned and supportive parents, she worked hard and was very successful academically, and she immersed herself in enjoyable, absorbing activities with various friends. She could exist in this world of light, sustained by a whole array of ties to others that were uncontaminated by the events of the darkness. When night came, however, everything was different: The caring father of the daylight disappeared as a strange leering grin came across his features and the sexual exploitation began. During the "special times," she felt erased, obliterated, turned into a thing. A means of enduring these deadly moments, as she later recalled it, was to watch the moon out of the corner of her eye, losing herself in its illuminated face until her father had finished with her. This reliance seemed to be reflected during the period of her later psychosis in a persistent delusional belief that the moon was a conscious entity that was following her and watching over her protectively.

The split between the patient's experience of the day and the night closely mirrored a division in the being of her father, who himself alternated between two sharply contrasting states: the state of being a normal parent to his daughter and that of being a leering sexual abuser with strange fantasies about love and ancient royalty. A second chronically recurring dream of the patient's childhood years expressed the tension created by these two fathers and by the separated worlds in which they carried on their distinctive activities. In this nightmare, the patient was lying prostrate and unclothed on the ground. On each side of her body were six or seven small men, like elves or gnomes, and each was holding a piece of string. On the end of each string was a hook, inserted into the patient's skin. At first, the line of elves on the right began to pull on their strings, stretching the patient's skin and pulling it outward, and then the row of little men on the left began pulling their strings and hooks, so that the patient's skin was pulled alternatingly first to the right, then to the left, then back to the right, and so on, until finally she would awaken in terror and confusion.

Let us now return to our initial question: What is the most important difference between traumatic experiences leading to annihilation and those that lead to the lesser reaction of dissociation? The circumstances that were the context of the patient's breakdown as a young woman amounted to a threefold attack on the normal world, itself protected by an enduring dissociation, that had sustained her throughout her life. She had lost the supportive social framework of her school years, her mother was being ravaged by cancer, and she had been violently assaulted by the physical environment in her car accident. In view of these losses, we can perhaps understand the enormous significance attaching to her call for help to her mother on the day of her collapse and the devastating effect of her mother's obliterating, invalidating response to that plea. That invalidation, occurring at a moment of extreme vulnerability, specifically recapitulated the reactions of both parents during her childhood when she expressed any need in relation to the massive abuse she was undergoing.

The trauma that annihilates subverts the person's whole way of making sense of his or her life and attacks sustaining connections to the human surround at their most fundamental level; the trauma that can be dissociated, although also a threat to existing organizations of experience, leaves sustaining ties intact to some degree, so that a stable platform of selfhood and worldhood survives for the encapsulation and dissociation of the traumatic event. In the clinical case just described, a relatively steady dissociation of the daylight and nighttime worlds was possible because of the very stability of that daylight sphere, and the annihilation experiences only commenced when the world of normality itself began to disintegrate. The specific triggering event preceding the patient's breakdown was the response of her mother to her request for help. This request was not only rebuffed but was redefined as having no foundation when the mother cheerfully reminded her daughter that she was perfectly capable of taking care of herself. The very structure of the patient's desperate effort to reach out to her family for something to rescue her was thus undercut, and the felt reality of her universe began accordingly to dissolve. The hallucination repeating the message, "You see . . . you're blind . . . you see . . . you're blind . . . ," crystallized this dissolution in an auditory form.

Very often there are no dramatic, easily identifiable events immediately preceding the advent of self- and world disintegration, and this can lead the Cartesian observer to conclude that the patient's psychosis is arising from wholly internal factors and processes. Such a conclusion, relying on crude distinctions between endogenous and exogenous psychopathology, fails to take into account the unique meanings that seemingly ordinary or even trivial occurrences may take on in the intersubjective field to which they belong. This context sometimes includes profound, ongoing issues of world formation tracing back to the vicissitudes of early life, issues touching on the person's very capacity to experience "I am." The flow of everyday happenings, no single aspect of which appears remarkable to the outside observer, may become relentlessly traumatic in relation to such issues, progressively stripping away sustaining connections to others and undermining the person's sense of his or her own existence. Sudden breakdowns without a provoking cause, gradual deteriorations in the absence of significant trauma and stress, unexplained eruptions of psychotic experience that can have no other source than a pathological process located inside the patient—these are among the phenomena that appear with compelling clarity under the lens of Cartesian understanding. A post-Cartesian viewpoint, by contrast, allows us to focus on the embeddedness of these psychological catastrophes in transactional, intersubjective fields. Such a focus often opens our eyes to previously unseen meanings in the patient's expressions, meanings in terms of which the manifestations of the so-called psychosis suddenly become newly intelligible. Most important, in the light of these revised understandings, new opportunities for therapeutic intervention also appear, and the devastation of the patient's world perhaps itself opens up to healing transformation.

References

Aron, L. 1996. *A meeting of minds: Mutuality in psycho-analysis.* Hillsdale, NJ: Analytic Press.

Atwood, G. E., and R. D. Stolorow. 1980. Psychoana-lytic concepts and the representational world. *Psychoanalysis and Contemporary Thought* 3:267–290.

_____. 1984. *Structures of subjectivity: Explorations in psychoanalytic phenomenology.* Hillsdale, NJ: Analytic Press.

_____. 1993. *Faces in a cloud: Intersubjectivity in per-sonality theory.* 2nd ed. Northvale, NJ: Jason Aronson.

Bacal, H., and K. Newman. 1990. *Theories of object rela-tions: Bridges to self psychology.* New York: Columbia University Press.

Bader, M. 1998. Postmodern epistemology: The prob-lem of validation and the retreat from therapeutics in psychoanalysis. *Psychoanalytic Dialogues* 8:1–32.

Beebe, B., and F. M. Lachmann. 1994. Representation and internalization in infancy: Three principles of salience. *Psychoanalytic Psychology* 11:127–165.

Beebe, B., F. M. Lachmann, and J. Jaffe. 1997. Mother-infant interaction structures and presymbolic self- and object representations. *Psychoanalytic Dialogues* 7:133–182.

Benjamin, J. 1995. *Like subjects, love objects: Essays on recognition and sexual difference.* New Haven, CT: Yale University Press.

_____. 1998. *Shadow of the other: Intersubjectivity and gender in psychoanalysis.* New York and London: Routledge.

Bergson, H. 1960. *Time and free will.* Translated by F. Pogson. New York: Harper Torchbooks. Original edition 1910.

Bernstein, R. 1983. *Beyond objectivism and relativism.* Philadelphia: University of Pennsylvania Press.

Bion, W. 1977. *Seven servants.* Northvale, NJ: Jason Aronson.

Bleichmar, H. 1999. A modular approach to the complexity of unconscious processes: Implications for psychoanalytic psychotherapy. Paper presented at the Institute for Psychoanalytic Self Psychology and Relational Psychoanalysis, Rome, March.

Brandchaft, B. 1994. To free the spirit from its cell. In R. D. Stolorow, G. E. Atwood, and B. Brandchaft, eds., *The intersubjective perspective*, pp. 57–76. Northvale, NJ: Jason Aronson. Original article 1993.

Brentano, F. 1973. *Psychologie vom empirischen standpunkte* (Psychology from an empirical standpoint). Leipzig/London: Felix Meiner/Routledge. Original edition 1874.

Brothers, L. 1997. *Friday's footprint: How society shapes the mind*. New York and Oxford: Oxford University Press.

Cavell, M. 1991. The subject of mind. *International Journal of Psycho-Analysis* 72:141–153.

———. 1993. *The psychoanalytic mind: From Freud to philosophy*. Cambridge: Harvard University Press.

Cilliers, P. 1998. *Complexity and postmodernism*. London and New York: Routledge.

Coburn, W. J. 2001. Subjectivity, emotional resonance, and the sense of the real. *Psychoanalytic Psychology* 18:303–319.

Cottingham, J., R. Stoothof, D. Murdoch, and A. Kenny, eds. and trans. 1991. *The philosophical writings of Descartes*. Vol. 3, *The correspondence*. Cambridge: Cambridge University Press.

Culler, J. 1982. *On deconstruction*. Ithaca, NY: Cornell University Press.

Davidson, R., and N. Fox. 1982. Asymmetrical brain activity discriminates between positive versus negative affective stimuli in human infants. *Science* 218:1235–1237.

Demos, E. V., and S. Kaplan. 1986. Motivation and affect reconsidered. *Psychoanalysis and Contemporary Thought* 9:147–221.

Derrida, J. 1978. *Writing and difference*. Translated by A. Bass. Chicago: University of Chicago Press.

Des Lauriers, A. M. 1962. *The experience of reality in childhood schizophrenia*. Madison, CT: International Universities Press.

Descartes, R. 1989a. *Discourse on method*. Buffalo, NY: Prometheus Books. Original edition 1637.

_____. 1989b. *Meditations.* Buffalo, NY: Prometheus Books. Original edition 1641.

Dilthey, W. 1989. *Introduction to the human sciences.* Translated by M. Neville et al. Princeton: Princeton University Press. Original edition 1883.

Duke, P., and G. Hochman. 1992. *A brilliant madness.* New York: Bantam Books.

Fairbairn, W. R. D. 1952. *Psychoanalytic studies of the personality.* London: Routledge and Kegan Paul.

Federn, P. 1952. *Ego psychology and the psychoses.* Edited by E. Weiss. New York: Basic Books.

Fosshage, J. L. 1989. The developmental function of dreaming mentation: Clinical implications. In A. Goldberg, ed., *Dimensions of self experience: Progress in self psychology,* vol. 5, pp. 3–11. Hillsdale, NJ: Analytic Press.

Frank, M. 1991. *Selbstbewusstsein und selbsterkenntnis* (Self-consciousness and self-knowledge). Stuttgart, Germany: Reclam.

_____. 1992. *Stil in der philosophie* (Style in philosophy). Stuttgart, Germany: Reclam.

Freud, S. 1953. The interpretation of dreams. In J. Strachey, ed. and trans., *The standard edition of the complete psychological works of Sigmund Freud,* vols. 4 and 5, pp. 1–627. London: Hogarth Press. Original edition 1900.

_____. 1957. The unconscious. In J. Strachey, ed. and trans., *The standard edition of the complete psychological works of Sigmund Freud,* vol. 14, pp. 159–215. London: Hogarth Press. Original article 1915.

_____. 1961a. The ego and the id. In J. Strachey, ed. and trans., *The standard edition of the complete psycho-*

logical works of Sigmund Freud, vol. 19, pp. 3–66.
London: Hogarth Press. Original edition 1923.

_____. 1961b. The loss of reality in neurosis and psychosis. In J. Strachey, ed. and trans., *The standard edition of the complete psychological works of Sigmund Freud,* vol. 19, pp. 183–187. London: Hogarth Press. Original article 1924.

_____. 1961c. Neurosis and psychosis. In J. Strachey, ed. and trans., *The standard edition of the complete psychological works of Sigmund Freud,* vol. 19, pp. 149–153. London: Hogarth Press. Original article 1924.

_____. 1964. New introductory lectures on psychoanalysis. In J. Strachey, ed. and trans., *The standard edition of the complete psychological works of Sigmund Freud,* vol. 22, pp. 1–182. London: Hogarth Press. Original edition 1933.

Friedman, L. 1999. Why is reality a troubling concept? *Journal of the American Psychoanalytic Association* 47:401–425.

Fromm-Reichman, F. 1954. An intensive study of twelve cases of manic-depressive psychosis. In *Psychoanalysis and psychotherapy: Selected papers,* pp. 227–274. Chicago: University of Chicago Press.

Gadamer, H.-G. 1991. *Truth and method.* 2nd ed. Translated by J. Weinsheimer and D. Marshall. New York: Crossroads. Original edition 1975.

Gaukroger, S. 1995. *Descartes: An intellectual biography.* Oxford: Oxford University Press.

Gendlin, E. T. 1988. *Befindlichkeit: Heidegger and the philosophy of psychology.* In K. Hoeller, ed., *Heidegger and Psychology,* pp. 43–71. Seattle: *Review of Existential Psychology and Psychiatry.*

Gerson, S. 1995. The analyst's subjectivity and the relational unconscious. Paper presented at the spring meeting of the Division of Psychoanalysis, American Psychological Association, Santa Monica, California.

Ghent, E. 1992. Foreword. In N. J. Skolnick and S. C. Warshaw, eds., *Relational perspectives in psychoanalysis,* pp. xiii–xxii. Hillsdale, NJ: Analytic Press.

Gill, M. M. 1982. *Analysis of transference.* Vol. 1. Madison, CT: International Universities Press.

———. 1994. Heinz Kohut's self psychology. In A. Goldberg, ed., *A decade of progress: Progress in self psychology,* vol. 10, pp. 197–211. Hillsdale, NJ: Analytic Press.

Gump, J. 2000. Social reality as an aspect of subjectivity: Outing race in the therapeutic space. Paper presented at the conference Motivation and Spontaneity: Celebration in Honor of Joseph D. Lichtenberg, M.D., Washington, DC, October.

Habermas, J. 1987. *Knowledge and human interests.* Translated by J. Shapiro. Cambridge: Polity Press. Original edition 1971.

Hamilton, V. 1993. Truth and reality in psychoanalytic discourse. *International Journal of Psycho-Analysis* 74:63–79.

Hegel, G. 1977. *The phenomenology of spirit.* Translated by A. Miller. Oxford: Oxford University Press. Original edition 1807.

Heidegger, M. 1962. *Being and time.* Translated by J. Macquarrie and E. Robinson. New York: Harper and Row. Original edition 1927.

Herman, J. 1992. *Trauma and recovery*. New York: Basic Books.

Hoffman, I. Z. 1983. The patient as interpreter of the analyst's experience. *Contemporary Psychoanalysis* 19:389–422.

Husserl, E. 1962. *Ideas: An introduction to pure phenomenology*. Translated by W. B. Gibson. New York: Collier. Original edition 1931.

_____. 1970. *The crisis of European sciences and transcendental phenomenology*. Translated by D. Carr. Evanston, IL: Northwestern University Press. Original edition 1936.

James, W. 1975. Philosophical conceptions and practical results. In *Pragmatism*. Cambridge: Harvard University Press. Original article 1898.

Jamison, K. R. 1995. *An unquiet mind*. New York: Alfred A. Knopf.

Jones, J. 1995. *Affects as process*. Hillsdale, NJ: Analytic Press.

Jung, C. G. 1965. The psychology of dementia praecox. In *The psychogenesis of mental disease: The collected works of C. G. Jung*, vol. 3, pp. 1–152. New York: Bollingen Foundation. Original edition 1907.

Kernberg, O. F. 1975. *Borderline conditions and pathological narcissism*. Northvale, NJ: Jason Aronson.

_____. 1976. *Object relations theory and clinical psychoanalysis*. Northvale, NJ: Jason Aronson.

Klein, M. 1950a. A contribution to the psychogenesis of manic-depressive states. In *Contributions to psychoanalysis 1921–1945*, pp. 282–310. London: Hogarth Press. Original article 1934.

_____. 1950b. *Contributions to psycho-analysis 1921–1945.* London: Hogarth Press.

Kohut, H. 1971. *The analysis of the self.* Madison, CT: International Universities Press.

_____. 1977. *The restoration of the self.* Madison, CT: International Universities Press.

_____. 1978. Introspection, empathy, and psychoanalysis. In P. Ornstein, ed., *The search for the self,* vol. 1, pp. 205–232. Madison, CT: International Universities Press. Original article 1959.

_____. 1980. Reflections on advances in self psychology. In A. Goldberg, ed., *Advances in self psychology,* pp. 473–554. Madison, CT: International Universities Press.

_____. 1982. Introspection, empathy, and the semicircle of mental health. *International Journal of Psycho-Analysis* 63:395–407.

_____. 1984. *How does analysis cure?* Edited by A. Goldberg and P. Stepansky. Chicago: University of Chicago Press.

_____. 1991. *The search for the self.* Vol. 4. Edited by P. Ornstein. Madison, CT: International Universities Press.

Laing, R. D. 1959. *The divided self.* London: Tavistock Publications.

Leary, K. 1994. Psychoanalytic "problems" and postmodern "solutions." *Psychoanalytic Quarterly* 63:433–465.

Leider, R. 1990. Transference: Truth and consequences. In A. Goldberg, ed., *The realities of transference: Progress in self psychology,* vol. 6, pp. 11–22. Hillsdale, NJ: Analytic Press.

Lichtenberg, J. 1989. *Psychoanalysis and motivation.*
Hillsdale, NJ: Analytic Press.

Lyotard, J.-F. 1984. *The postmodern condition: A report on knowledge.* Manchester, England: Manchester University Press.

Margulies, A. 2000. Commentary. *Journal of the American Psychoanalytic Association* 48:72–79.

Maroda, K. 1991. *The power of countertransference.* Northvale, NJ: Jason Aronson.

May, R., E. Angel, and H. Ellenberger, eds. 1958. *Existence.* New York: Basic Books.

Merleau-Ponty, M. 1962. *The phenomenology of perception.* New York: Humanities Press. Original edition 1945.

Mitchell, S. A. 1988. *Relational concepts in psychoanalysis: An integration.* Cambridge: Harvard University Press.

Nagel, T. 1986. *The view from nowhere.* New York and Oxford: Oxford University Press.

Nietzsche, F. 1973. *Beyond good and evil.* Harmondsworth and New York: Penguin Books. Original edition 1886.

Ogden, T. 1994. *Subjects of analysis.* Northvale, NJ: Jason Aronson.

Orange, D. M. 1995. *Emotional understanding: Studies in psychoanalytic epistemology.* New York: Guilford Press.

———. 1996. A philosophical inquiry into the concept of desire in psychoanalysis. *Psychoanalysis and Psychotherapy* 13:122–129.

———. 2000. Book review of *The Chicago Institute lectures* by H. Kohut. *Psychoanalytic Psychology* 17:420–431.

———. 2002a. Antidotes and alternatives: Perspectival realism and the new reductionism. *Psychoanalytic Psychology* 19: in press.

_____. 2002b. There is no outside: Empathy and authenticity in psychoanalytic process. *Psychoanalytic Psychology* 19: in press.

_____. 2002c. Why language matters to psychoanalysis. *Psychoanalytic Dialogues* 12: in press.

Orange, D. M., G. E. Atwood, and R. D. Stolorow. 1997. *Working intersubjectively: Contextualism in psychoanalytic practice.* Hillsdale, NJ: Analytic Press.

Peirce, C. 1878. How to make our ideas clear. *Popular Science Monthly* 12:286–302.

_____. 1931–1935. *The collected papers of Charles Sanders Peirce.* Edited by C. Hartshorne and P. Weiss. Cambridge: Harvard University Press. Original edition 1905.

Piaget, J. 1974. *The place of the sciences of man in the system of sciences.* New York: Harper and Row. Original edition 1970.

Putnam, H. 1990. *Realism with a human face.* Cambridge: Harvard University Press.

Renik, O. 1993. Analytic interaction: Conceptualizing technique in light of the analyst's irreducible subjectivity. *Psychoanalytic Quarterly* 62:553–571.

_____. 1999. Remarks. Commentary given at the PEP CD-ROM Symposium on the Analytic Hour: Good, Bad, and Ugly, New York, February.

Rorty, R. 1989. *Contingency, irony, and solidarity.* Cambridge: Cambridge University Press.

Sander, L. 1985. Toward a logic of organization in psychobiological development. In H. Klar and L. Siever, eds., *Biologic Response Styles,* pp. 20–36. Washington, DC: American Psychiatric Association.

Sandler, J., and B. Rosenblatt. 1962. The concept of the representational world. *The Psychoanalytic Study of the Child* 17:128–145.

Sands, S. 1997. Self psychology and projective identification—Whither shall they meet? *Psychoanalytic Dialogues* 7:651–668.

Schafer, R. 1972. Internalization: Process or fantasy? *The Psychoanalytic Study of the Child* 27:411–436.

Scharfstein, B. 1980. *The philosophers: Their lives and the nature of their thought.* Oxford: Oxford University Press.

Schutz, A. 1970. *Reflections on the problem of relevance.* New Haven: Yale University Press.

Searles, H. 1965. *Collected papers on schizophrenia and related subjects.* London: Hogarth Press.

Shane, M., E. Shane, and M. Gales. 1997. *Intimate attachments: Toward a new self psychology.* New York: Guilford Press.

Siegel, D. J. 1999. *The developing mind.* New York: Guilford Press.

Slavin, M. 2002. Post-Cartesian thinking and the dialectic of doubt and belief in the treatment relationship. *Psychoanalytic Psychology* 19:307–323.

Socarides, D. D., and R. D. Stolorow. 1984–1985. Affects and selfobjects. *Annual of Psychoanalysis* 12/13:105–119.

Stern, D. B. 1997. *Unformulated experience: From dissociation to imagination in psychoanalysis.* Hillsdale, NJ: Analytic Press.

Stern, D. N. 1985. *The interpersonal world of the infant.* New York: Basic Books.

Stern, S. 1994. Needed relationships and repeated relationships: An integrated relational perspective.
Psychoanalytic Dialogues 4:317–349.

Stolorow, R. D. 1974. A neurotic character structure built
upon the denial of an early object loss. Graduation
paper, Psychoanalytic Institute of the Postgraduate
Center for Mental Health, New York.

_____. 1990. The world according to whom? In A.
Goldberg, ed., *The realities of transference: Progress in
self psychology,* vol. 6, pp. 35–40. Hillsdale, NJ: Analytic
Press.

_____. 1994. The nature and therapeutic action of psy-
choanalytic interpretation. In R. D. Stolorow, G. E.
Atwood, and B. Brandchaft, eds., *The intersubjective
perspective,* pp. 43–55. Northvale, NJ: Jason Aronson.
Original article 1993.

_____. 1997. Dynamic, dyadic, intersubjective systems:
An evolving paradigm for psychoanalysis. *Psychoanalytic
Psychology* 14:337–346.

_____. 1999. The phenomenology of trauma and the
absolutisms of everyday life: A personal journey.
Psychoanalytic Psychology 16:464–468.

Stolorow, R. D., and G. E. Atwood. 1979. *Faces in a
cloud: Subjectivity in personality theory.* Northvale, NJ:
Jason Aronson.

_____. 1989. The unconscious and unconscious fantasy:
An intersubjective-developmental perspective.
Psychoanalytic Inquiry 9:364–374.

_____. 1992. *Contexts of being: The intersubjective founda-
tions of psychological life.* Hillsdale, NJ: Analytic Press.

_____. 1997. Deconstructing the myth of the neutral analyst: An alternative from intersubjective systems theory. *Psychoanalytic Quarterly* 66:431–449.

Stolorow, R. D., G. E. Atwood, and B. Brandchaft. 1994. Epilogue. In R. D. Stolorow, G. E. Atwood, and B. Brandchaft, eds., *The intersubjective perspective*, pp. 203–209. Northvale, NJ: Jason Aronson.

Stolorow, R. D., G. E. Atwood, and J. M. Ross. 1978. The representational world in psychoanalytic therapy. *International Review of Psycho-Analysis* 5:247–256.

Stolorow, R. D., B. Brandchaft, and G. E. Atwood. 1987. *Psychoanalytic treatment: An intersubjective approach.* Hillsdale, NJ: Analytic Press.

Stolorow, R. D., and F. M. Lachmann. 1975. Early object loss and denial: Developmental considerations. *Psychoanalytic Quarterly* 44:596–611.

Sucharov, M. 1994. Psychoanalysis, self psychology, and intersubjectivity. In R. D. Stolorow, G. E. Atwood, and B. Brandchaft, eds., *The intersubjective perspective*, pp. 187–202. Northvale, NJ: Jason Aronson.

Sullivan, H. S. 1950. The illusion of personal individuality. *Psychiatry* 13:317–332.

_____. 1953. *The interpersonal theory of psychiatry.* New York: Norton.

Tausk, V. 1917. On the origin of the influencing machine in schizophrenia. *Psychoanalytic Quarterly* 2:519–556.

Taylor, C. 1989. *Sources of the self: The making of the modern identity.* Cambridge: Harvard University Press.

Thelen, E. 1989. Self-organization in developmental processes: Can systems approaches work? In M. Gunnar and E. Thelen, eds., *Systems in development:*

The Minnesota symposia in child psychology, vol. 22, pp. 77–117. Hillsdale, NJ: Lawrence Erlbaum Associates.

Thelen, E., and L. Smith. 1994. *A dynamic systems approach to the development of cognition and action.* Cambridge: MIT Press.

Toulmin, S. 1990. *Cosmopolis.* Chicago: University of Chicago Press.

Wasserman, M. 1999. The impact of psychoanalytic theory and a two-person psychology on the empathizing analyst. *International Journal of Psycho-Analysis* 80:449–464.

Winnicott, D. W. 1958a. *Collected papers: Through paediatrics to psychoanalysis.* New York: Basic Books.

_____. 1958b. The manic defense. In *Collected papers: Through paediatrics to psychoanalysis,* pp. 129–144. New York: Basic Books. Original article 1935.

_____. 1965. *The maturational processes and the facilitating environment.* Madison, CT: International Universities Press.

_____. 1971. The use of an object and relating through identifications. In *Playing and reality,* pp. 86–94. New York: Basic Books. Original article 1969.

Wittgenstein, L. 1953. *Philosophical investigations.* New York: Macmillan.

_____. 1958. *The blue and brown books: Preliminary studies for the "philosophical investigations."* New York: Harper and Row.

_____. 1961. *Tractatus logico-philosophicus.* Atlantic Highlands, NJ: Humanities Press. Original edition 1921.

Zeddies, T. 2000. Within, outside, and in between: The relational unconscious. *Psychoanalytic Psychology* 17:467–487.

Index